Plant Based Diet.

A Beginner Guidebook Loaded with Powerful Natural Vegetables, Fruits, whole grains, Legumes, Nuts and Seeds for a Healthier Lifestyle and Irrevocable Weight Loss.

HELEN KINGSLEY

DEDICATION

To all who desire to live life to the fullest!

TABLE OF CONTENT

INTRODUCTION..1

PROCEDURES TO EATING TO LOSE WEIGHT BASED ON A PLANT WHOLE DIET 2

Breakfast 9

Banana with Peanut Butter Oats 9

White Bean Toast with Avocado...............................10

Parfait Peach Pie Breakfast 12

Mango Almond Vegan Milkshake 13

Avocado and Spinach Vegan Smoothie 14

Mocha Espresso with Peanut Butter Shake 15

Vegan Banana smash Oatmeal 16

Banana and Chocolate Chip Pancakes 17

Peanut Butter Bar 19

Breakfast Quinoa & blueberries................................20

Breakfast Quickie 23

Overnight Banana Walnut-Oatmeal 23

Slow Cooked Chocolatey Pistachio Oatmeal.............24

Chilled Oatmeal with Bananas & Berries 25

Slow Cooked Pumpkin & Cranberry Granola 27

Pumpkin Pie Pudding with Chia Seeds......................28

Blueberry Chia Seed with Honey Pudding 30

Yogurt Parfait Breakfast Recipe 31

Peanut Buttered with Berries Toast...........................32

Easy Avocado & Feta Toast 33

Veggie Muffins & Egg..34

Apple and Pumpkin Muffin Recipe 35

Zero Baked Workout Bars..37

Vegan Quinoa Protein Bars.......................................38

Slow Cooked Steel-Cut Oatmeal with vanilla............40

Overnight Slow Cooked Pumpkin Pie with Oats-Zero
Sugar 41

Savory Mexican Slow Cooked Oats 43

Lunch 45

Chickpeas-Kale Salad with Maple Dijon Dressing 45

Paleo Mango & Black Bean Tacos 47

Potatoes stuffed with Wild Rice and Herbs Recipe...48

Butternut Squash with Cranberry Salad 50

Pumpkin Chili 52

Avocado Hummus Dish..53

Fusion Burritos..55

Oil-Free Salad Dressing Recipes 57

Red Lentil and Butternut Squash Stew 59

Spicy Butternut Squash Soup Recipe 61

Butternut Mash Soup with Apple & Thyme.............62

Butternut Squash and Spinach Lasagna...................64

Simple Butternut Tacos...67

Creamy Butternut With Squash Soup 69

Dinner & Side Dish 71

Potato Salad with Plant-Based Mayonnaise 71

Plant Based Chili Recipe..73

Maple Glazed Tempeh with Quinoa, Kale and Garlic75

Lentil Vegetable Loaf 77

Mushroom and Broccoli Stir-Fry Formula................79

White Bean Stew 81

Quinoa Vegan Meat Recipe 83

Black Bean Lentil Soup 85

Greek Lentil and Garlic Soup....................................86

Quinoa Lentil and Mustard Burger 89

Grilled Spicy Tofu with Szechuan Veggies.................91

Cleansing Vegetable Soup..93

Snacks 97

Easy To Make Stuffed Mushrooms Formula.............97

Plant-Based- Cashew Bread 99

Limed Cilantro With Three Bean Salad 100

Chia-Spiced Candied Nuts 102

Vegan Avocado Wontons..103

Vegan Sunflower Lentil Dip.......................................105

Quinoa and Lentils Meatballs 106

Spicy Mango Salsa...109

Spinach and Artichoke Dip Recipe 110

Chocolate and Peanut Butter Bites...........................112

Desserts 115

Banana Pudding Cream...115

Avocado and Banana Brownie Formula...................116

Vegan No-Bake Cookie chocolate coated dough Bars

....117

Vegetarian Caramel Apple Parfait............................119

Spiced Carrot Oatmeal Cookies 121

Peppermint Fudge Formula 122

Nutty Banana Chocolate Bread.................................124

Lemony Cranberry Cheesecake-Vegan 126

Coconut and Mango Ice Cream 128

Vegan Strawberry Banana Bread..............................129

Oil-Free chocolate Muffin Recipe 130

Smoothies 133

Avocado and Pear Smoothie.....................................133

Blue Paradise and Pineapple Smoothie 134

Super Smoothie 135

Super Blast Smoothie..136

Immune Booster Vegan Smoothie 137

Ever-young Smoothie..138

Banana Ginger and Pomegranate Mishmash 139

Quinoa Raspberry Smoothie...................................140

Peanut Butter Cum Banana Mishmash...................141

Mediterranean Organic Smoothie............................142

Sunrise Smoothie 143

Strawberry and Goji Berry Cumbo 145

Minty Blueberry and Flax Seed Smoothie...............146

Mango & Basil Smoothie...147

Skinny Banana Split Protein Smoothie....................148

Mango and Orange Smoothie Diet...........................149

Vegan Pumpkin Spice Smoothie 150

Apple and Coconut Smoothie 151

Razzle-Dazzle Smoothie-Vegan...............................152

INTRODUCTION

A Pant-based-diet is a diet consisting classically of foods obtained from plants. It has more of a spotlight on eating whole, unprocessed foods.

Such foods including grains, vegetables, nuts, legumes, seeds, and fruits, and with a little or no animal products

Legumes and further plant-based proteins (like soybeans and seitan)

Whole grains which includes oats, quinoa and brown rice.

Good fats, such as avocados

Greens – and as much as possible!

Maple syrup, coconut sugar, and other unrefined sugars (stay away from artificial sweeteners)

Nuts and seeds, including nut milk, chia seeds, flax seeds

Natural starches, such as potatoes

Coffee is inclusive

Fruits and veggies

PROCEDURES TO EATING TO LOSE WEIGHT BASED ON A PLANT WHOLE DIET

Plant based weight loss

There are numerous aspects that could be part of the cause to weight loss, the most popular one being exercise. And, yes, exercise is indispensable. You must be actively moving your body regularly in order to lose excess body fat.

I have to let you know categorically that exercise is not the only thing that could make you lose body fats, if you can exercise all you like, and you replenish those lost calories with fatty convenience foods you likely won't divest yourself of the extra weight. Now the question is; what else can I do with exercise to lose weight promptly?

As you've in all probability heard by now, going plant-based can do a lot of incredulity for your health and weight loss. When you live a plant-based life, you can do things excessive exercise can't do. A plant-based lifestyle will provide you with a sustainable lifestyle that can maintain the weight loss in longer term than every other diet.

Here in this book, you will learn how to eat well to lose weight effectively longer and still live a healthy lifestyle without any form of hassle.

Now that sounds simple enough, but what does it really signify? And most especially, how can you put it into practice?

There are some general principles to follow for your weight loss to be effective; this includes adjusting things as you go so as to be in tune with your weight loss needs & proclivity.

These procedures will aid you a great deal in achieving the body you so desire;

1. Eat whole plant foods:

This means restraining processed foods made from flours and refined ingredients. For example, choose bananas or apples over fruit juices; brown over white rice; chickpeas or sweet potatoes over pasta or crackers. Plant foods in their whole form have more nutrients than you can ever imagine and it will do your body a lot of favor to eating processed and canned foods.

2. Concentrate on nutrient-density:

With a higher vitamin and mineral content, raw fruits and vegetables are the healthiest foods you can eat. On account of their greater volume, water, and nutrition content, they fill you up and leave you more contented after each meal.

Whole nutrients-dense foods such as legumes, veggies, whole grains and fruits are foods that should frame the better part of your diet. One thing these foods have in common is fewer calories, more nutrients which is exactly what your body needs. Long term continual weight loss, requires satisfaction. This is the more reason why nutrient dense foods should be your focus.

3. Be S.O.S free:

Steer clear of sugar, oil and salt and especially oil because it adds-in more than necessary calories while salt and sugar then again promotes overindulging.

Aside the fact they make you stuff yourself unnecessarily, they don't hold any nutritional advantage and the lesser sugar, oil and salt you eat, the lesser your body will crave them. If you are worried about low intake of sodium, never worry because you can get it from whole natural foods.

A better way to have an SOS- free diet, is preparing your own home-made savory vegetable broth liquid, you can mix-in, in your meals, when you cook.

4. Keep all deliberate (overt) fats in check:

The basic rule, to drop weight when on a plant whole based diet is to munch on lower fat (especially oil) and protein (also, lower your seeds, avocado, and nuts & other fatty foods ingestion). For starters, maintain about 10% (or even lesser) of calories from fat and 15% from protein. Centre your meals on vegetables, legumes, whole grains and fruits. To eat clean, take seeds, nuts more as a condiment than the major calorie constituents of the brunch. You can add-in coconut recipes or sauces in your diet, but don't make it an everyday thing.

5. Maintain hydration:

Drink water (over beverages) every morning and during the day because more than half your body is water and needs replenishing. Exercise and digestion necessitate a lot of water and after hours with zero food and fluid, your body's water needs refilling. Eating lots of vegetables, raw fruits and zero salt will also keep your body hydrated.

6. **Do not under-eat:**

You need to have an estimated view of the amount of calories you need to consume, so you can eat as much as necessary. A calorie shortage is always needed to lose weight but if you under-eat, you will not keep with it for long and may end up overindulging. Tools like the chronometer can provide you with a general idea of the wide ranging amount of calories your food holds and this is very important, most especially if you are a very active person. Losing fat should not be your main concern but also building & maintaining muscles.

7. **Be consistent:**

Do whatever drives you and stick with it. Find a eating pattern, you can stick with, daily or weekly; not eating well for a couple of weeks then skimping off, the next 2 weeks, so to say, then climbing back on again, not a good approach. Mold your food choices to fit in your way of life. you can even create a meal plan, and plan your meal weekly (in batch), set in meal prep containers. Basically, just stick to what you can.

8. **Well organized meal prep is the answer:**

Batch cooking is a good way to go; setting up your food in advance will help, especially on busier nights. Spend less time on thinking about food to prepare, start by making meals that do not take long to prepare and maybe few of your favorite recipes and the more you familiarize yourself in cooking them, the less time you will feel is required to work on them.

9. Keep eating simple:

Keeping it simple is deciding on a few meals you prefer, and eating them frequently this can aid in weight loss (repeating it) most especially when your body is transitioning and also help improve healthy eating habits. Avoid additives and stimulating food that will push you to eat more than needed. This includes oil, sugar, and salt and yes, spices. Eating simple will re-set your body, so that you eat not because you want to eat but because you are hungry.

10. Apply attentiveness:

Avoid multi-tasking while eating, if not you will eat more than necessary, and miss the signs that your body does not need anymore. Pay more attention so you can enjoy the flavors of the food and also stop eating, when you need to stop. The simpler and cleaner you eat, and the more attentive you are when eating, the more in sync with these signs, you will be.

11. Enjoy your food:

You can look forward to your meals, by picking out/choosing foods and recipes you enjoy. Do not be afraid to try out new recipes.

Whole plant based foods are the best foods you can feed your body with and also one of the beneficial food that is nourishing and also aids to lose weight and maintain it.

Whole plant foods can help you create a lifestyle that promotes healthy living with nutrient dense, whole foods that may stretch to every areas of your life.

So build up a healthy eating habits by following the principles above to lose that added weight, and maintain it long term!.

Breakfast

Banana with Peanut Butter Oats

Prep Time: 10 mins

Total Time: 10 min

Serve: 2 cups

Nutrition:

Calories: 227; Fiber: 5 g; Total Fat: 11 g; Protein: 7 g; Sodium: 47 mg; Cholesterol: 0 mg; Saturated Fat: 2 g; Sugar: 9 g; Trans Fat: 0 g;

Constituents:

1/2 tsp cinnamon (ground)

1/2 cup rolled oats

1 tbsp chia seeds

Almond milk (1 cup)

Chia seeds (1 tbsp)

1 tbsp honey (vegan option: maple syrup)

Vanilla extracts (1/4 tsp)

1 banana, sliced

2 tbsps natural creamy peanut butter

Methods:

1: Combine the oats, cinnamon, milk and honey together and mix well.

2: Pour a small portion into 2 jars or any serving containers.

3: Layer with the sliced banana and peanut butter.

4. Finish with the remaining mixture on top.

5: Seal and cover the containers and allow sitting overnight. Best served chilled.

White Bean Toast with Avocado

Prep Time: 11 min

Total Time: 11 min

Serves: 5

Nutrition:

Calories: 140; Fiber: 5g| Carbs: 19g| Total Fat: 5g| Cholesterol: 0mg| Protein: 6g| Trans Fat: 0g| Saturated Fat: 1g| Sodium: 212mg| Sugar: 2g|

Constituents:

Kosher salt (1/2 tsp)

White beans, canned (1/2 cup; rinsed and drained)

1/4 cup grape tomatoes, halved

2 tsps Tahini paste

2 tsps lemon juice

Avocado, (half; pit removed and peeled)

4 slices whole bread (or your favorite) toasted

Methods:

1. In a bowl, Tote up the beans, Tahini, 1 tsp lemon juice and half the salt. Mash it well

2. In another bowl, lightly mash the beans, remaining lemon juice and salt.

3. Pick up your toast and spread the mashed beans first, spread the avocado on top and finish with the tomatoes. Serve

Parfait Peach Pie Breakfast

Prep Time: 7 min

Total Time: 7 min

Serve: 4; Size: 1 cup

Nutrition:

Calories: 260 | Fiber: 8g| Saturated Fat: 4g| Total Fat: 13g
Carbohydrates: 30g| Sodium: 20mg| Protein: 6g| Trans
Fat: 0g | Sugar: 13g| Cholesterol: 0mg

Constituents:

1/4 cup chia seeds

1/2 cup granola

1 tbsp pure maple syrup

1 cup coconut milk

3 medium peaches (diced to small size)

1 tsp ground cinnamon

Methods:

1. In a bowl, Mix the chia seeds, coconut milk and maple syrup.

2. Cover the mixture and refrigerate for one hour.

3. Tote up the cinnamon and diced peaches. Set it aside

4. Divide the chia mixture into two jars or glasses. Top each jar with granola, reserving two spoons

5. Divide the peach mixture equally between the jars and finish with the granola that was reserved. Serve

Mango Almond Vegan Milkshake

Prep Time: 7 min

Total Time: 7 min

Serve: 1; Size: 1 smoothie

Nutrition:

Calories: 228; Carbs: 51 g| Fiber: 7 g| Sodium: 131 mg| Total Fat: 3 g| Saturated Fat: 1 g| Protein: 4 g| Sugars: 44 g| Cholesterol: 0 mg| Trans Fat: 0 g |

Constituents:

1 ripe mango (pulp)

3/4 cup (unsweetened) almond milk

Ice cubes

Instructions:

1. In a blender, put all Constituents and blend it until smooth

Drink immediately.

Avocado and Spinach Vegan Smoothie

Prep Time: 5 min

Total Time: 5 min

Quota: 2; Quota Size: 1 3/4 Cup

Nutrition:

Calories: 299; | Total Fat: 19 g | Fiber: 8 g| Cholesterol: 18 mg| Protein: 11 g| Saturated Fat: 5 g| Carb: 24 g| Sodium: 75 mg| Sugars: 13 g

Constituents:

1/2 cup spinach

2 tbsps honey, Agave nectar or any natural sweetener

2 cups almond milk, chilled

Ice cubes

1 avocado

Methods:

1. Put all constituents in a blender and blend until smooth.

2. Serve cold

Mocha Espresso with Peanut Butter Shake

Prep Time: 5 min

Total Time: 5 min

Quota: 1;

Nutrition:

Calories: 179; Carbs: 21 g| Sodium: 97 mg| Total Fat: 10 g| Cholesterol: 0 mg| Protein: 6 g| Sugar: 9 g| Fiber: 6 g

Constituents:

1/2 frozen banana

1/2 cup almond milk

1 tbsp peanut butter

Cocoa powder, unsweetened (1 tbsp)

1/2 cup almond milk

Strong brewed coffee, chilled (1/2 cup)

3/4 cup ice cube

Methods:

1. Pour all the constituents into a blender

2. Pound until becomes smooth

Vegan Banana smash Oatmeal

Prep Total: 12 Mins

Total Time: 12 Mins

Serves: 1

Nutrition: Calories: 217; Carbs: 46g| Fiber: 7g| Sodium: 98mg| Total Fat: 3g| Saturated Fat: 1g| Trans Fat: 0g| Protein: 5g Cholesterol: 0mg| Sugar: 17g|

Constituents:

1/4 cup oats

1/4 tsp cinnamon

1/2 cup almond milk, unsweetened

1 recipe Roasted Banana Smash

Methods:

1. Make the Roasted Banana Smash recipe.

2. In a pot, Tote up the other Constituents and allow boiling.

3. Reduce the heat and allow cooking for another 5 min.

4. Set the pot down and Tote up the roasted banana smash. Serve

Banana and Chocolate Chip Pancakes

Prep Time: 10 min

Cook Time: 30 min

Total Time: 40 min

Serve: 6 pancakes; Serve Size: 1 pancake

Nutrition:

Calories: 271; Protein: 5g| Fiber: 4g| Total Fat: 16g|
Trans Fat: 0g| Saturated Fat: 13g| Carbohydrates: 32g|
Sugar: 7g Cholesterol: 0mg| Sodium: 218mg

Constituents:

3 tbsps melted coconut oil

1 cup coconut milk

2 tbsps coconut sugar

1 large overly ripe banana, (mashed)

1 1/2 cups whole wheat flour

1 tsp baking soda

1/2 cup vegan chocolate chips

Methods:

1. Tote up the sugar, oil, milk and banana in a clean bowl. Mix well.

2. Stir in the flour and baking soda carefully. Be sure not to over mix.

3. Fold in chocolate chips carefully.

4. Spray a large skillet with a non-stick spray and place on medium heat.

5. Pour 1/4 of the batter into the skillet and cook for 4 min.

6. Flip and cook the other side for another 3 min.

7. Remove pancake from heat once ready and cook the remaining batter in the same way.

8. Remember to grease the skillet with the spray in-between the cooking.

9. Serve pancakes hot and drizzle with honey, coconut butter, fruit, and maple syrup if desired.

Peanut Butter Bar

Prep Time: 15 min

Cook Time: 1 hour

Total Time: 1 hour 15 min

Quota: 8; Quota Size: 1 bar

Nutrition:

Calories: 232; Fiber: 4g| Cholesterol: 0mg| Total Fat: 9g|
Sugar: 30g| Carbs: 39g| Saturated Fat: 2g | Protein: 5g|
Sodium: 3mg| Trans Fat: 0g

Constituents:

1 cup oats (cooked)

1 1/2 cups date (pit removed)

1/2 cup peanut butter

Methods:

1. Line a baking pan with parchment paper.

2. In a food processor, put the dates and roughly chop.

3. After chopping the dates, Tote up the oats and peanut
butter. Blend until just combined.

4. Pour and press the mixture into the prepared sheet and
keep in the refrigerator for duration of 1 hour.

5. Cut up and serve.

Breakfast Quinoa & blueberries

Prep Time: 10 min

Cook Time: 20 min

Total Time: 30 min

Quota: 1

Nutrition:

Calories: 326; Protein: 8g| Cholesterol: 0mg| Total Fat: 6g |Trans Fat: 0g| Fiber: 6g| Saturated Fat: 1g| Sugar: 28g Carbohydrates: 64g| Sodium: 192mg

Constituents:

1/2 cup fresh blueberries

1/4 cup coarsely chopped walnuts

1 banana, (peeled and sliced)

1/2 cup quinoa, (pre-rinsed)

1/8 tsp salt

2 tbsps honey, raw preferred

1/2 cup milk (or almond milk)

Methods:

1. To a saucepan, Tote up 1 cup of water, quinoa and salt. Bring the water to boil and reduce the heat.

2. Cook for 15 min.

3. Beat with a fork and Tote up the milk and honey.

4. Divide the mixture in an even way between two bowls and Tote up banana slices, nuts and almond milk as toppings.

Breakfast Quickie

Overnight Banana Walnut-Oatmeal

Prep Time: 5 min

Total Time: 5 min

Serve: 2

Calories: 213; Fiber: 3g| Sodium: 117mg| Sugar: 28g| Total Fat: 5g| Cholesterol: 6mg| Trans Fat: 0g| Protein: 7g| Saturated Fat: 1g| Carbohydrates: 38g

Constituents:

Oats:

1/3 cup rolled oats

1/2 cup low-fat milk

1/3 cup plain low-fat yogurt

1 tbsp honey

1/4 tsp ground cinnamon

1/4 tsp vanilla extract

a pinch of sea salt

The Serving:

1/4 cup chopped walnuts

1 banana, peeled and sliced

Methods:

1. In two bowls, Tote up all the Constituents, stir and cover. Refrigerate for 7 hours.

2. Serve chilled or heat in a microwave. Tote up banana slices and walnuts as toppings.

Slow Cooked Chocolatey Pistachio Oatmeal

Prep Time: 10 min

Cook Time: 1 hour 30 min

Total Time: 1 hour 40 min

Serve: 4; Serve Size: 3/4 Cup

Calories: 254; Fiber: 6 g| Sodium: 2 mg| Protein: 9 g| Total Fat: 12 g| Sugars: 1 g| Saturated Fat: 2 g | Carbohydrates: 30 g| Trans Fat: 0 g | Cholesterol: 0 mg|

Constituents:

2 tbsps cocoa powder

4 tbsps crushed pistachios (divided)

1 cup steel-cut oats

5 cups water

Oil (for coating)

2 tbsps coconut sugar

Methods:

1. Coat the slow cooker with oil to prevent oats from sticking.

2. Into the cooker, Tote up the water, cocoa powder, oats, sugar and half the pistachios.

3. Cook on low for 90 min. Stir before serving and sprinkle with the remaining pistachios and low fat milk (optional).

Chilled Oatmeal with Bananas & Berries
Prep Time: 10 min

Total Time: 10 min

Serve: 2

Nutrition:

Calories: 236; Fiber: 7g| Trans Fat: 0g| Total Fat: 9g| Cholesterol: 5mg| Sodium: 49mg| Saturated Fat: 3g| Protein: 8g| Sugar: 14g| Carbohydrates: 33g|s

Constituents:

1/4 cup Greek yogurt

1/4 cup old-fashioned oats

1 banana, (peeled and sliced)

Almond milk (1/3 cup)

1 tbsp honey, (raw)

1/2 tsp (real) vanilla extract

Chia seeds (1 tbsp)

1/2 cup fresh raspberries

2 tbsps shredded coconut, (unsweetened)

1/4 cup orange juice

1/4 tsp ground cinnamon

2 half-pint jars

Methods:

1. In a bowl, combine the Constituents except the orange juice, and coconut berries and banana slices.

2. Pour a part of the oat mixture into a jar. Tote up the banana slices and orange juice to prevent them from becoming brown.

3. Top with oat mixture, banana slices and half of the berries.

4. Replicate the process in another jar. Cover it and keep in the freezer overnight.

Slow Cooked Pumpkin & Cranberry Granola

Prep Time: 15 min

Cook Time: 2 hours

Total Time: 2 hours 15 mins

Serve: 24

Calories: 223 | Fiber: 5 g| Saturated Fat: 5 g| Total Fat: 10 g | Sugars: 5 g| Sodium: 2 mg| Cholesterol: 0 mg| Protein: 7 g| Trans Fat: 0 g | Carbohydrates: 29 g

Constituents:

1/4 cup sliced almonds

1/4 cup ground flax seed

1/2 cup coconut oil

1/4 cup honey

5 cups rolled oats

1/4 cup pumpkin seeds

1/4 cup chopped pecans

1 tsp pure vanilla extract

2 tsps pumpkin pie spice

1/2 cup dried cranberries

Methods:

1. To your slow cooker, Tote up all the ingredients and stir until the coconut oil is melted.

2. Leaving the lid slightly open, cook on low setting for 2 hours. Stir twice.

3. Remove and allow cooling totally.

Pumpkin Pie Pudding with Chia Seeds

Prep Time: 7 min

Total Time: 7 min

Serve: 4

Nutrition:

Calories: 252; Sodium: 34mg| Trans Fat: 0g| Sugar: 10g| Total Fat: 16g | Cholesterol: 0mg| Protein: 5g| Carbs: 24g| Saturated Fat: 1g| Fiber: 10g

Constituents:

2 cups canned coconut milk

1 cup pumpkin puree

1/4 cup coconut sugar

1/4 tsp all spice

1/2 cup of chia seeds

4 tbsps whipped topping, (optional)

1 tsp cinnamon

1/2 tsp ginger

1/2 tsp nutmeg

Methods:

1. Blend all the Constituents leaving the chia seed. Blend until it is smooth.

2. Tote up the chia seed and pulse until it is well combined.

3. Clean dessert dishes and divide the batter. Close the lid and place in the refrigerator overnight. Tote up whipped topping if desired when serving.

Blueberry Chia Seed with Honey Pudding

Prep Time: 10 min

Total Time: 10 min

Serve: 4

Nutrition:

Calories: 172; Cholesterol: 0 mg| Fiber: 6 g| Total Fat: 6 g
Carbohydrates: 26 g| Saturated Fat: 1 g| Trans Fat: 0g|
Sodium: 61 mg| Protein: 4 g| Sugars: 17 g|

Constituents:

1/2 tsp vanilla extract

1 cup blueberries

1/4 cup granola for topping (optional)

1 1/2 cups almond milk (or coconut milk)

1/2 cup chia seeds

Methods:

1. In a food processor, puree all the Constituents except
the chia seeds.

2. Stir in the chia seeds.

3. Pour mixture into individual cups and refrigerate
overnight. A thick pudding consistency should be
achieved.

Yogurt Parfait Breakfast Recipe

Prep Time: 10 min

Total Time: 10 min

Serve: 3

Nutrition:

Calories: 184; Protein: 6 g| Fiber: 4 g| Total Fat: 8 g |
Trans Fats: 0 g| Sugars: 1 g| Saturated Fats: 4 g| Carbs:
23 g| Sodium: 35 mg| Cholesterol: 0 mg|

Constituents:

1/4 cup (unsweetened, shredded) coconut

1/2 cup granola

1 cup grapes or mixed berries

1/2 banana, (chopped)

1/2 cup non-fat yogurt

Methods:

1. In a clean jar, lay grapes or berries, Tote up another
layer of yogurt, then granola, fruit, yogurt again and
shredded coconut. Cover the lid.

Peanut Buttered with Berries Toast.

Prep Time: 5 min

Total Time: 5 min

Serve: 4

Calories: 204; Protein: 7 g| Fiber: 4 g| Sugars: 4 g|
Cholesterol: 0 mg| Total Fat: 9 g | Carbohydrates: 25 g|
Trans Fat: 0 g| Sodium: 175 mg| Saturated Fat: 2 g

Constituents:

4 slices whole grain or whole wheat toast

4 tbsps sugar free (or homemade) peanut butter

1 cup raspberries, or blackberries, or both

Methods:

1. Spread out the peanut butter in an even way on toast
and Tote up berries as toppings on each toast.

Easy Avocado & Feta Toast

Prep Time: 5 min

Cook Time: 5 min

Total Time: 10 min

Serve: 2

Nutrition: Calories: 297: Protein: 9g| Cholesterol: 22mg| Total Fat: 21g| Fiber: 8g| Saturated Fat: 6g | Carbs: 22g| Trans Fat: 0g | Sugar: 3g| Sodium: 364mg

Constituents:

1 ripe avocado, (peeled and pitted)

2 slices whole wheat bread

Crumbled feta cheese (1/3 cup)

Methods:

1. Toast the bread slices to taste.

2. In a bowl, mash avocado with a potato masher until it gives a creamy consistency.

3. On each toast, spread the milky avocado and finish with feta cheese.

Veggie Muffins & Egg

Prep Time: 10 min

Cook Time: 20 min

Total Time: 30 min

Serve: 6

Calories: 118; Carbs: 2g| Fiber: 1g| Sugar: 1g| Total Fat: 8g| Protein: 9g| Saturated Fat: 3g | Sodium: 328mg| Trans Fat: 0g | Cholesterol: 196mg

Constituents:

6 large eggs

1/2 tsp kosher or sea salt

1/4 tsp black pepper

1/2 cup grated cheddar cheese

1/2 red bell pepper (diced)

1 cup diced zucchini

1/4 cup diced onion

Methods:

1. Set oven to 375 degrees.

2. Get a 6-cup tin for regular sized muffins and oil lightly.

3. In a bowl, beat the Constituents except cheese until it is fluffy.

4. Fill 3/4 of each muffin cup with the batter. Sprinkle cheese onto each cup. Bake in the oven for 20 mins.

Apple and Pumpkin Muffin Recipe

Prep Time: 10 min

Cook Time: 15 min

Total Time: 25 min

Serve: 8

Nutrition:

Calories: 149 | Fiber: 4g | Sugars: 5g | Sodium: 264 mg | Protein: 4g | Total Fat: 10 g| Carbohydrates: 11g | Cholesterol: 82 mg

Constituents:

4 eggs

1 tsp baking soda

2 tsps vanilla

4 tbsps coconut oil

2 tbsps cinnamon

1/4 tsp ground cloves

1/2 cup applesauce

1/2 cup pureed pumpkin

1/2 cup coconut flour

1/4 tsp ground ginger

1/8 tsp ground nutmeg

1/4 tsp sea salt

Methods:

1. Set oven to 375 degrees.

2. Clean muffin tins and line it.

3. Blend all Constituents in a blender on low speed until it just combine.

4. Divide the batter into 8 tins. Cook in the oven for the duration of 15 min. Allow to cool and serve.

Zero Baked Workout Bars

Prep Time: 15 min

Total Time: 15 min

Serve: 12 bars

Calories: 333; Fiber: 5 g| Trans Fats: 0 g| Carbohydrates: 37 g| Total Fat: 18 g| Protein: 14 g| Sodium: 14 mg| Saturated Fats: 6 g| | Sugars: 19 g| Cholesterol: 1 mg

Constituents:

1 cup natural peanut butter

1/2 cup lite coconut milk,

1/4 cup honey (raw honey if possible)

1/2 cup mini chocolate chips

1/2 cup chia seeds (or ground flax seeds)

1/2 cup raisins

2 cups rolled oats

1/2 cup protein powder

Methods:

1. Pulse 1 1/2 cups of oats until it becomes flour in a blender.

2. Combine the oat flour, remaining oat, chocolate chips, raisins and chia or flax seed. Toss well.

3. Stir the coconut milk, honey and peanut butter in another clean bowl. Pour into the oat mixture.

4. Stir thoroughly and spread into a 9 x 9 inch square pan.

5. Press down in the pan and cover with a foil. Refrigerate until it hardens.

6. Cut into 12 bars and enjoy.

Vegan Quinoa Protein Bars

Prep Time: 20 mins

Cook Time: 2hrs 20 mins

Total Time: 40 min

Serve: 8 bars

Nutrition:

Calories: 376; Fiber: 10 g| Trans Fats: 0 g| Total Fat: 13 g | Saturated Fats: 3 g | Sugars: 33 g | Carbohydrates: 63 g Cholesterol: 0 mg| Sodium: 3 mg| Protein: 14 g

Constituents:

1/2 cup raw almonds with skin

1/3 cup almond butter

Chocolate chips (1/4 cup)

1 tbsp honey (optional)

Quinoa, (1/3 cup; pre-rinsed)

Water (2/3 cup)

16 whole (pitted) dates

Methods:

1. In a sauce pan, Tote up water and quinoa and allow boiling. Reduce heat and allow simmering for the duration of 14 min.

2. Allow cooked quinoa to cool and keep in the refrigerator overnight or for the duration of 2 hours.

3. In a blender, Tote up the dates and pulse till it forms a ball. Remove and position in a mixing bowl'

4. Pulse the almonds until it is finely minced.

5. Tote up peanut butter, chilled quinoa and dates to the almonds in the blender and pulse until well combined.

6. Pour mixture into a mixing bowl and mould into six bars.

7. Melt the honey and the chocolate chips in a sauce pan over low heat.

8. On each bar, spread a thin layer of the melted chocolate. Refrigerate the bars and allow them to become hard.

Slow Cooked Steel-Cut Oatmeal with vanilla

Prep Time: 10 min

Cook Time: 2 hours

Total Time: 2 hours 10 min

Serve: 4

Nutrition:

Calories: 126; Fiber: 2.1 g| Sugars: 4.4 g| Trans Fat: 0g| Sodium: 160 mg| Total Fat: 8 g | Carbs: 12.4 g| Saturated Fat: 6.4 g | Protein: 2.7 g| Cholesterol: 0 mgs

Constituents:

1 tbsp cocoa powder

1 tsp vanilla

1 cup steel-cut oats

4 cup water

1/2 cup coconut milk

1/4 tsp salt

1 tbsp coconut palm sugar (or pure maple syrup)

8 drops stevia, liquid (or an extra tbsp of sugar)

Methods:

1. Combine milk, water, stevia and vanilla in a clean bowl. Tote up cocoa, salt and sugar. Beat.

2. Tote up your oats.

3. Oil the slow cook to prevent oatmeal from sticking.

4. Pour in the mixture and cook on low for 2 hours.

5. Keep cooker on warm before bed. Give it a stir in the morning before serving.

6. Top with chocolate (optional).

Overnight Slow Cooked Pumpkin Pie with Oats-Zero Sugar

Prep Time: 2 min

Cook Time: 8 hours

Total Time: 8 hours 2 min

Serve: 4

Nutrition Info:

Calories: 188; Cholesterol: 0 mg| Fiber: 2 g| Total Fat: 1 g
| Saturated Fat: 0 g | Protein: 1 g| Carbs: 15 g| Trans Fat:
0 g | Sugars: 7 g| Sodium: 193 mg

Constituents:

1 tsp vanilla extract

1/4 tsp salt

1 tsp pumpkin pie spice

Oats, steel cut (1 cup)

3 cups water (or almond or milk)

Canned pumpkin puree (1 cup)

Methods:

1. Tote up all Constituents into the slow cooker.

2. Cook on low heat for 8 hours.

Savory Mexican Slow Cooked Oats

Prep Time: 5 min

Cook Time: 3 hours

Total Time: 3 hours 5 min

Serves: 4

Calories: 159; Protein: 8 g| Fiber: 5 g| Total Fat: 3 g|
Carbohydrates: 29 g| Trans Fat: 0 g| Sugars: 5 g| Sodium:
507 mg| Cholesterol: 0 mg| Saturated Fat: 1 g

Constituents:

2 tbsps fresh cilantro, (chopped)

2 cups low-sodium chicken broth, (no sugar)

1 cup salsa

1 cup steel cut oats

1 cup frozen corn, (thawed)

1 cup red pepper, (chopped)

Methods:

1. Tote up all Constituents in the slow cooker. Cover.

2. Cook for 3 hours.

44

Lunch

Chickpeas-Kale Salad with Maple Dijon Dressing

Prep Time: 12 mins

Total Time: 12 mins

Quota: 3

Nutritional Info:

Calories: 294; Sugar: 18g| Cholesterol: 0mg| Fiber: 15g| Total Fat: 5g| Saturated Fat: 0g| Protein: 14g| Trans Fat: 0g | Carbs: 52g| Sodium: 447mg

Constituents:

Salad:

3 cups kale, (roughly chopped)

1/2 cup carrot, (shredded)

15 ounce canned chickpeas, (well-drained and rinsed)

1/2 tsp cayenne pepper

1/4 tsp red pepper flakes

1 jalapeno pepper, (sliced thinly)

1/2 cup red onion, (sliced thinly)

Dressing:

1 tbsp Dijon mustard

1 tsp orange zest

1/4 cup apple cider vinegar

2 tbsps pure maple syrup

Methods:

1. Tote up the chick peas, red pepper flakes and chickpeas in a large bowl. Toss well.

2. In a larger bowl, pour the chickpeas mixture and Tote up the remaining salad Constituents. Toss well and dish into serving bowls.

3. Top with 3 tsps of dressing. Serve.

 Dressing:

1. Tote up the Constituents for the dressing and beat well. Allow to sit for about 5 min.

2. Before you tote up the salad, give dressing a stir.

Paleo Mango & Black Bean Tacos

Prep Time: 12 mins

Cook Time: 15 mins

Total Time: 27 mins

Serves: 3

Nutritional Info:

Calories: 420; Fiber: 20g| Sodium: 543mg| Total Fat: 12g|
Saturated Fat: 2g| Protein: 14g| Sugar: 18g| Trans Fat: 0g
| Cholesterol: 0mg| Carbohydrates: 70gs

Constituents:

1/4 cup vegetable broth

6 gluten free corn tortillas

1 ripe mango, (sliced into strips)

1 avocado, pit and peel removed, (cut into small chunks)

2 Roma tomatoes, (diced)

2 tbsps red onion, (diced)

1/4 cup orange bell pepper, (diced)

1 tbsp lime juice

2 tbsps fresh cilantro, (diced)

1/2 tsp Kosher salt

15 ounce canned black beans, (well-drained and rinsed)

Methods:

1. Mix the bell pepper, cilantro, lime juice, tomatoes, onions and salt in a large bowl. Cover bowl and keep aside.

2. Heat the vegetable broth and beans in a pot. Allow to simmer for 5 min.

3. Remove pot from heat and mash the content lightly. Mixture should be chunky.

4. On high heat, place a skillet and heat. When hot, Tote up a corn tortilla. Cook until brown. Flip and cook the other side.

5. When brown, remove and cook the remaining. Place in a warm plate.

6. On a clean flat surface, spread the tortillas and layer with the black beans mixture.

7. Top with avocado and mango.

8. Finish with the tomato mixture. Serve.

Potatoes stuffed with Wild Rice and Herbs Recipe

Prep Time: 20 min

Cook Time: 1 hour 30 min

Total Time: 1 hour 50 min

Serve: 4

Nutritional Info:

Calories: 360; Protein: 11 g| Carbohydrates: 65 g| Total
Fat: 8 g | Sodium: 281 mg| Saturated Fat: 1 g | Fiber: 8g
Sugars: 4 g| Trans Fat: 0 g| Cholesterol: 0 mg|

Constituents:

2 tbsps sparsely (fresh chopped)

2 tbsps basil (fresh chopped)

2 tbsps olive oil, (divided)

1/2 tsp coarse sea salt, (divided)

1 shallot, (minced)

1 clove garlic, (minced)

4 cups baby spinach

1 cup wild rice, (cooked according to package Methods)

1 tbsp lemon juice, (fresh)

1/4 tsp ground black pepper, (fresh)

1 tsp minced chives

4 large russet potatoes

Methods:

1. Set oven to 350 degrees.

2. Coat half of the russet potatoes in half tbsp of oil and rub the other half of the potatoes with salt.

3. Place potatoes in a baking sheet and bake for 30 min.

4. While baking the potatoes, place a skillet over medium heat and pour the remaining oil.

5. Cook the garlic and shallots in the oil until tender. Tote up spinach and cook until it is wilted.

6. Tote up the cooked rice and remove skillet from heat. Tote up the lemon juice, herbs and salt and pepper.

7. When potatoes are done, cut each along the middle.

8. Stuff with half cup of the rice mixture and serve.

Butternut Squash with Cranberry Salad

Prep Time: 5 min

Cook Time: 5 min

Total Time: 10 min

Serve: 4

Nutrition Info:

Calories: 327; Fiber: 5 g| Cholesterol: 0 mg| Total Fat: 20 g | Sugars: 4 g| Protein: 6 g| Carbs: 33 g| Saturated Fat: 3 g| Sodium: 11 mg

Constituents:

5 tbsps extra-virgin olive oil

2 cups cooked quinoa

1/2 cup dried cranberries

3 cups butternut squash (diced)

1/3 cup walnuts pieces

1 tbsp basil (freshly chopped)

1/4 tsp sea salt

1/4 tsp black pepper

Methods:

1. Place a sauce pan on medium heat. Tote up 3 tbsps of extra-virgin olive oil and sauté the squash until soft.

2. Mix the cooked squash and all other Constituents and the remaining 2 tbsps of olive oil. Serve.

Pumpkin Chili

Prep Time: 15 min

Cook Time: 6 hours

Total Time: 6 hours 15 min

Serve: 6 cups

Nutrition Info:

Calories: 214; Fiber: 16g| Sugar: 11g| Cholesterol: 0mg|
Total Fat: 1g| Saturated Fat: 0g| Sodium: 841mg| Protein:
12g| Trans Fat: 0g | Carbohydrates: 43g|

Constituents:

1 jalapeno, (veins and seeds removed and minced)

Garlic, minced (2 cloves)

1 onion, (diced)

 Drained black beans, 2 (14 oz) cans

1 carrot, (shredded)

1 (diced) bell pepper,

1 onion, (diced)

Crushed tomatoes- 2 (14 oz) cans

1 1/2 cups pumpkin puree

Vegetable broth, low-sodium (1 cup)

2 tbsps chili powder

1 tsp pumpkin pie spice

Kosher salt (1 tsp)

1/2 tsp black pepper

Methods:

1. To the slow cooker, Tote up all the Constituents and stir well.

2. Cook over low heat for the duration of 6 hours.

3. Top with avocado slices or a dollop of Greek yogurt when serving

Avocado Hummus Dish

Prep Time: 10 min

Total Time: 10 min

Serve: 4

Nutrition Info:

Calories: 196; Cholesterol: 0mg| Protein: 8g| Total Fat: 6g| Saturated Fat: 1g | Carbohydrates: 29g| Trans Fat: 0g | Fiber: 7g| Sodium: 275mg| Sugar: 9g|

Constituents:

15-ounce canned chickpeas, (drained and rinsed)

1/2 medium sized cucumber, (sliced thinly)

1/2 ripe avocado, (peeled, pitted, and sliced thickly)

10 spinach leaves

1/3 cup clean eating hummus, (home-made or store-bought, any variety)

1 cup baby carrots

2/3 cup grape tomatoes

2 tbsps pumpkin or shelled sunflower seeds, optional

1/4 tsp kosher or sea salt

1/4 tsp black pepper

Methods:

1. Layer a clean bowl with the spinach leaves.

2. To one corner, Tote up avocado slices, to other corner grape tomatoes, chickpea to another corner and to the last corner baby carrots.

3. To the middle of the bowl, Tote up humus and top it with pumpkin seeds or sunflower (optional).

4. Sprinkle with salt and pepper to taste.

Fusion Burritos

Prep Time: 30 minutes

Total Time: 30 minutes

Serve: 18 burritos

Nutrition Info:

Calories: 397; Fiber: 7g| Protein: 11g| Sugar: 7g| Total Fat: 9g| Carbohydrates: 71g| Sodium: 170mg| Saturated Fat: 1g| Trans Fat: 0g| Cholesterol: 0mg|ss

Constituents:

18 rice paper wrappers

5 ounces mixed baby greens, (organic if possible)

16 ounce package firm or super firm block of tofu

Vegan oil-free salad dressing (your choice)

2 bell peppers, (any color)

2 cups shredded carrots

2 cups shredded purple cabbage

8 ounces brown rice noodles

1 avocado

1 cucumber

Methods:

1. Prepare the rice noodles.

2. Peel the avocado, slice the avocado, bell peppers and cucumber into wide strips.

3. Prepare the tofu without the marinade and slice into wide strips.

4. In a big bowl, Tote up all the vegetable fillings and the oil free salad dressing.

5. Toss well and coat the vegetables.

6. Prepare the rolls by dipping each sheet of rice wrapper in temperate water for 10 secs. Place wrappers on a clean work surface.

7. Scoop the vegetable filling across the lower third of the wrapper and leave space on the sides.

8. Place an even amount of the tofu and rice noodles over the vegetable filling and fold over the edges of the burritos into tubes.

9. Place the rolls on a tray.

Oil-Free Salad Dressing Recipes

Prep Time: 5 minutes

Total Time: 5 minutes

Serve: 4

Nutrition Info:

Recipes under 50 Calories per serve

Constituents:

Tamari Vinaigrette Recipe:

1/4 cup tamari

1/4 cup balsamic (or red wine vinegar)

1001 Islands:

6 tbsps silken tofu

3 tbsps stone ground mustard

3 tbsps ketchup

1 tsp freshly squeezed lemon juice

Pinch of salt

Pinch of freshly ground pepper

Agave Mustard Recipe:

1/4 cup stone ground mustard

2 tsps Dijon mustard

1/4 cup silken tofu

3 tbsps agave syrup

Salt

Pinch of freshly ground black pepper

Strawberry Vinaigrette:

4 large strawberries

2 tbsps agave syrup

1 tbsp red wine vinegar

pinch of freshly ground black pepper

Creamy Italian Recipe:

6 tbsps soft silken tofu

2 tsps fresh squeezed lemon juice

4 tbsps water

1/2 tsps each garlic powder, onion powder, oregano flakes, rosemary flakes, basil flakes, and salt

Pinch of freshly ground black pepper

Sesame umami Recipe:

2 tbsps toasted sesame seeds

1/4 cup tamari or soy sauce

1 large clove garlic (finely crushed)

2 tbsps rice vinegar

2 tbsps water

Methods:

1. For the tamari vinaigrette, beat the tamari and mix with the salad.

2. To prepare the 1001 Islands dressing, puree all the Constituents in a blender.

3. To make the agave mustard, place all Constituents in a blender and puree.

4. Mix all Constituents for strawberry vinaigrette in a food processor and puree.

5. Puree tofu and water in a food processor then blend in other Constituents to retain its color from herb flakes for the creamy Italian.

6. In a skillet, toast sesame seeds over medium heat until they pop. Grind seeds and combine well with all other dressings.

Red Lentil and Butternut Squash Stew
Prep Time: 15 mins

Cook Time: 8 hrs

Total Time: 8hrs 15 mins

Serve: 4

Nutrition Info:

Calories: 227; Fiber: 18 g| Trans Fat: 0 g| Total Fat: 1 g |
Sodium: 101 mg| Carbs: 42 g| Saturated Fat: 0 g|
Cholesterol: 0 mg| Protein: 14 g| Sugars: 5 g

Constituents:

1 small onion, (diced)

3 stalks celery, (diced)

1 medium carrot, (diced)

1 tsp dried sage

1 tsp dried oregano

1 large butternut squash, (peeled and cubed)

1 cup red lentils (dried)

6 cups vegetable stock

Sea salt

Fresh ground pepper

Methods:

1. Tote up all the Constituents into the slow cooker.

2. Put lid on and cook for 7-8 hrs.

3. Dish up straight away

Spicy Butternut Squash Soup Recipe

Prep Time: 40 minutes

Total Time: 40 minutes

Serve: 16

Nutrition Info:

Calories: 146; Protein: 7 g| Trans Fat: 0 g| Total Fat: 3 g |
Sugar: 6| Sodium: 298 mg| Saturated Fat: 2 g| Fiber: 4 g|
Carbohydrates: 25 g| Cholesterol: 8 mg |

Constituents:

8 cups fat-free, low-sodium chicken broth

6 medium butternut squash, (seeded, halved and roasted
until tender)

2 cups plain 2% Greek yogurt

2 medium yellow onions, chopped

3 tbsps butter

1 tsp cumin

½ tsp coriander

½ tsp ginger

½ tsp marjoram

¼ tsp black pepper

¼ tsp cayenne pepper

Methods:

1. Set oven to 400 degrees.

2. Cut the ends and stems of the squash and half along its length. Place cut side on a lined baking sheet.

3. Roast for 50 min. Cool and scoop out flesh into a bowl.

4. Ina heavy bottom stockpot, heat butter, Tote up onions and cook till it is tender.

5. Tote up the peppers, coriander, cumin, ginger and marjoram and squash to the stockpot. Stir well and all it simmer for 20 min.

6. Place in a food processor and puree.

7. Pour back into the pot and simmer for Tote up for additional 20 min.

8. Tote up in the yogurt before serving

Butternut Mash Soup with Apple & Thyme
Prep Time: 10 min

Cook Time: 32 min

Total Time: 42 min

Quota: 4

Nutrition Info: Calories: 144; Fiber: 3.0 g| Trans Fat: 0 g| Carbs: 18.4g Total Fat: 7.9 g| Saturated Fat: 1.3 g| Protein: 2.5 g| Cholesterol: 2 mg | Sodium: 590 mg| Sugars: 9.0 g

Constituents:

24 ounces chicken stock

1 Granny Smith Apple, (peeled, cored, and diced)

2 tbsp olive oil

2 cups butternut squash, (diced)

2 tsp fresh thyme leaves

½ cup low-fat milk

1 clove garlic, (minced)

¼ tsp cumin

½ onion, diced

Salt

Pepper

Methods:

1. Over medium heat, heat olive oil in a pot and sauté the garlic and onion.

2. To the pot, Tote up the apple and squash. Stir well to coat. Cover the pot and reduce the heat.

3. Allow the vegetables to steam for 7 min. Check to make sure veggies are nit browning.

4. Tote up the thyme, cumin and stock to the pot and simmer for 25 min.

5. Pour into a food processor, Tote up milk and blend until puree.

Butternut Squash and Spinach Lasagna

Prep Time: 20 min

Cook Time: 4 hours

Total Time: 4 hours 20 min

Serve: 8

Nutritional info: Calories: 261; Fiber: 4.7 g| Cholesterol: 19 mg| Sugars: 2.6| Total Fat: 7.9 g | Carbs: 35.2 g| Saturated Fat: 3.5 g | Protein: 12.7| Trans Fat: 0 g | Sodium: 115 mg

Constituents:

Butternut squash puree Recipe:

2 cups of butternut squash, (chopped and minced)

1/2 medium yellow onion, (chopped)

1 shallot, (minced)

4 cloves of garlic, peeled, (chopped into 4)

1 tbsp extra virgin olive oil

4 fresh sage leaves (minced)

1/2 tsp of black pepper

1/2 tsp nutmeg

1/2 tsp ground rosemary

1/2 tsp ground thyme

Spinach Ricotta Muddle:

Whole grain uncooked lasagna pasta

4 cups of fresh spinach

1/2 tsp black pepper

15 oz container of part skim Ricotta

1/4 cup parmesan or asiago cheese, (pre mixed and shredded)

Methods:

1. Set the oven to 400 degrees.

2. Put the butternut, shallot, onion, sage leaves, thyme, rosemary, black pepper and extra virgin olive oil in a bowl and stir.

3. Pour on a cookie sheet and roast it for an hour. Take care to stir every 20 min.

4. Place the mixture in a food processor and blend into a puree.

5. Into a bowl, pour the puree and stir in nutmeg.

6. Mix the spinach, black pepper and ricotta in another bowl.

7. Clean your crock pot and spray with olive oil.

 How to layer your lasagna

1. Pour 1/3 of the puree into the Crockpot. Tote up paste to make a layer.

2. Top with another 1/3 of puree. Pour 1/2 of the spinach mixture and sprinkle with cheese.

3. Tote up a different stratum of pasta and pour the remaining butternut and spinach mixture.

4. Sprinkle with cheese.

5. Cook for 3 hours on low heat.

Simple Butternut Tacos

Prep Time: 15 min

Cook Time: 10 min

Total Time: 25 min

Serve: 4

Nutrition:

Calories: 327; Fiber: 8 g| Sodium: 113 mg| Total Fat: 20 g | Saturated Fat: 5 g| Sugars: 3 g| Trans Fat: 0 g| Protein: 8 g| Cholesterol: 13 mg| Carbs: 33 g|

Constituents:

1 cup butternut squash (lightly cooked)

1/2 tsp chipotle powder

4 corn tortillas

2 tbsps olive oil

1 cup lettuce (shredded)

1/2 cup cheese (shredded)

1 diced tomato (diced)

1 sliced avocado

1/2 tsp paprika

1/4 tsp onion powder

1/8 tsp garlic powder

1/8 tsp chili powder

Salt

Methods:

1. Cook the butternut squash,

2. with a fork, poke holes in the skin of the squash. Microwave for 3 min and remove carefully.

3. Peel the skin and cut into cubes.

4. In a bowl, mix all the seasonings and toss in the butternut cubes and coat.

5. Prepare taco shells or make use of purchased taco shells.

6. In a pan, warm 1tbsp oil and sauté the butternut cubes until its brown on the outside.

7. Spoon the squash into the taco shells and Tote up lettuce, avocado and tomato to garnish.

Creamy Butternut With Squash Soup

Prep Time: 10 mins

Cook Time: 41 mins

Total Time: 51 mins

Serve: 4

Nutritional Info:

Calories: 308; Sodium: 250 mg| Fiber: 5 g| Protein: 8 g
Total Fat: 17 g| Carbs: 33 g| Cholesterol: 2 mg| Saturated
Fat: 9 g| Trans Fat: 0 g| Sugars: 8 g

Constituents:

1 lb of squash, sliced

Onion, white (1 medium) and roughly chopped

4 cups of vegetable broth

Olive oil

Fresh thyme

1 tsp of grated nutmeg

Salt

Ground pepper

2/3 Cup of canned coconut milk (whole preferred)

Method:

1. Fry the onion, in a large sauté pan using olive oil and on medium heat for 3 mins.

2. After that, put-in the squash and heat for roughly 11 mins; stirring constantly.

3. Next, you Tote up-in the vegetable broth & boil on low for 20 mins.

4. Spice with pepper & salt and don't forget the nutmeg.

5. While the soup is still in the sauté pan, squash it, with an immersion blender.

6. After that, you Tote up-in the coconut milk, heat for 10 mins and then the thyme.

7. Turn off the fire and dish up while hot.

Dinner & Side Dish

Potato Salad with Plant-Based Mayonnaise

Prep Time: 10 min

Cook Time: 3 hours 35 min

Total Time: 3 hours 45 min

Serve: 6

Nutrition Info:

Calories: 124; Fiber: 3 g| Carbs: 27 g| Total Fat: 1 g|
Trans Fat: 0 g| Protein: 4 g| Saturated Fat: 0 g| Sodium:
612 mg| Sugar: 3 g| Cholesterol: 0 mg

Constituents:

2 pounds red potatoes, with skins

1 tbsp sea salt

1/2 cup (diced) celery

1/2 cup (diced) red onion

1/2 paprika (for garnish, optional)

Plant-Based Mayonnaise

Onion powder (1/2 tsp)

Sea salt (1 tsp)

1/2 tsp black pepper

1 cup raw cashews

Lemon juice, freshly squeezed (2 tbsps)

2 tbsps white wine vinegar

1 tsp garlic powder

3/4 cup water

2 tbsps Dijon mustard

2 tbsps whole-grain mustard

1/3 cup chopped dill weed

2 cups water for soaking

Methods:

1. Rinse the potatoes well and scrub. Cut into cubes.

2. To a big pot, Tote up the potatoes and 1 tbsp of salt, cover with water and boil.

3. Reduce heat and cook until tender. Drain, cover and keep aside.

4. In a big bowl, pour the cashew and Tote up 2 cups of water and allow sitting for the duration of 15 min. Drain and rinse.

5. Tote up the cashew to a blender, Tote up 3/4 cup of water and blend till a creamy consistency. Pour into a mixing bowl.

6. To the mixture, Tote up the other Constituents leaving the red onions and celery. Beat until combined.

7. To the potatoes. Tote up the red onions and celery, toss well.

8. Pour a cup of mayonnaise or as desired over the potatoes and toss well.

9. Salt and paprika can be Tote up if desired.

10. Cover the bowl and keep in the refrigerator for the duration of 3 hours before serving.

Plant Based Chili Recipe

Prep Time: 20 min

Cook Time: 9 hours

Total Time: 9 hours 20 min

Serve: 12 cups chili

Nutrition Info:

Calories: 216; Sugar: 6g| Sodium: 463mg| Fiber: 11g| Total Fat: 1g | Saturated Fat: 0g | Trans Fat: 0g| Cholesterol: 0mg| Carbohydrates: 41g| Trans Fat: 0g| Protein: 12g

Constituents:

1 tbsp chili powder

2 tbsps oregano flakes

1 tbsp cumin powder

3 cups dry pinto beans

3 bell peppers, red, yellow, and green, chopped

8 large green jalapeño peppers, (diced after removing seeds)

2 (14.5 ounce) cans of diced tomatoes

1 large yellow onion, (chopped)

Garlic powder (1 tbsp)

3 bay leaves, (freshly ground)

1 tsp ground black pepper

1 tbsp sea salt

Method:

1. Soak beans overnight. Drain and rinse the beans very well.

2. In a slow cooker, cook beams with 1 tbsp of salt for six hours on high setting.

3. After cooking, drain and mix in the other Constituents. Cook for another 3 hours.

4. Dish up with brown rice and adorn with avocado, salsa, red onions and fresh cut lime if desired.

Maple Glazed Tempeh with Quinoa, Kale and Garlic

Prep Time: 10 min

Cook Time: 15 min

Total Time: 25 min

Serve: 4

Nutrition Info:

Calories: 321; Sodium: 9 mg| Cholesterol: 0 mg| Total Fat: 12 g| Protein: 16 g| Saturated Fat: 2g | Sugars: 6 g| Trans Fat: 0 g | Fiber: 4 g| Carbs: 39 g|

Constituents:

1 tbsp fresh (chopped) thyme

1 tbsp fresh (chopped) rosemary

1 tbsp olive oil

1 1/2 cups vegetable stock

8 ounces tempeh, (cubed)

2 tbsps pure maple syrup

3 tbsps (dried) cranberries

1 clove garlic, (minced)

4 ounces baby kale, (chopped)

1 cup quinoa

Juice of 1 orange

Methods:

1. Heat oven to a temperature of 400 degrees.

2. Put the stock in a pot and allow boiling. Tote up quinoa.

3. Cover, reduce heat and allow simmering until it is fluffy and all liquid is absorbed.

4. Tote up the tempeh and maple syrup and put on a baking sheet that is covered with parchment paper.

5. Put sheet in the oven and bake for 15 min until the tempeh is brown in color and caramelized lightly.

6. While baking, Tote up the rest of the Constituents in a bowl. Tote up the tempeh and quinoa and incorporate well.

7. Tote up pepper with salt to taste.

Lentil Vegetable Loaf

Prep Time: 20 min

Cook Time: 45 min

Total Time: 1 hour 5 min

Serve: 6

Nutrition Info: Calories: 226; Sodium: 381mg | Total Fat: 6g | Protein: 12g Saturated Fat: 1g | Cholesterol: 0mg | Sugar: 8g | Trans Fat: 0g | Carbohydrates: 34g | Fiber: 9g

Constituents:

Ketchup Topping

1/3 cup ketchup

1 tsp balsamic vinegar

1 tsp Dijon mustard, (or yellow mustard)

Loaf Recipe

1/2 cup almond meal

1 1/2 tsps dried oregano

2 cups cooked lentils, (well-drained)

1 small onion, (diced)

1 carrot, (diced)

1 stalk celery, (diced)

8-ounce packaged white or button mushrooms, (cleaned and diced)

3 tbsps tomato paste

2 tbsps Liquid Amino, (or Tamari or gluten-free lite soy sauce)

Balsamic vinegar (1 tbsp)

Old-fashioned oats- 1 cup, uncooked (for gluten-free recipe, check the label)

Methods:

1. Heat the oven to a temperature of 400 degrees.

2. In a skillet, Tote up 1/4 water and onion. Sauté until it is soft. Tote up water as it evaporates.

3. Tote up carrot, mushrooms and the celery and keep sautéing until the mushrooms release its fluid. Drain and keep aside.

4. To a food processor, Tote up lentils, liquid amino, vinegar, tomato paste, oats, oregano and almond meal and blend until Constituents are well combined.

5. Pour mixture into a mixing bowl.

6. Tote up the mushrooms and vegetables to the food processor and blend until it is chunky. Tote up this to the mixing bowl.

7. Stir the mixture well.

8. Spray a loaf pan with a non-sticky cooking spray and Tote up the Constituents. Form into a loaf shape.

9. Bake in the oven for 35 min, Tote up the ketchup topping and bake for another 15 min.

10. Take away from the oven and allow resting for the duration of 10 min before you slice and serve it.

Mushroom and Broccoli Stir-Fry Formula

Prep Time: 12 minutes

Cook Time: 22 minutes

Total Time: 34 minutes

Serve: 4

Nutrition Info: Calories: 133; Fiber: 3g| Protein: 6g| Total Fat: 8g | Carbs: 12g| Saturated Fat: 1g| Sugar: 3g| Trans Fat: 0g| Sodium: 286mg| Cholesterol: 0mg|

Constituents:

1/4 tsp crushed red pepper (optional)

2 tsps fresh ginger, (grated)

2 cups broccoli, cut into small florets

1/4 cup red onion, chopped small

3 cloves garlic, minced

1/4 cup vegetable broth (or water)

1/2 cup carrot, (shredded)

1/4 cup cashews, (optional water chestnuts)

2 tbsps rice wine vinegar

Soy sauce, low-sodium (2 tbsps)

1 tbsp coconut sugar, (optional)

1 tbsp sesame seeds

2 cups mushrooms, (sliced)

Methods:

1. In a skillet on high heat, Tote up water, broccoli, red pepper, mushrooms and ginger.

2. Cook and stir often until the broccoli is tender.

3. Tote up broth as much as required to prevent the vegetables from sticking to the pan.

4. Tote up the carrot, soy sauce, cashew, and vinegar and coconut sugar if used and stir well. Simmer for 2 min.

5. Sprinkle the sesame seeds as toppings.

Serve alone or with quinoa or brown rice.

White Bean Stew

Prep Time: 5 min

Cook Time: 4 hours 30 mins

Total Time: 4 hours 35 min

Serve: 6

Nutritional Info: Calories: 238; Fiber: 10g | Total Fat: 4g | Carbs: 37g | Saturated Fat: 2g | Protein: 16g | Sodium: 809mg | Trans Fat: 0g | Cholesterol: 6mg | Sugar: 4g

Constituents:

30 ounces canned navy beans

1 large carrot (peeled and diced)

1/4 cup celery (diced)

1/2 cup yellow onion (diced)

3 cloves garlic (minced)

1/2 tsp red pepper (crushed)

1 tsp dried thyme

1 tsp dried oregano

1 tsp dried rosemary

2 1/2 cups low-sodium vegetable broth

14 ounce canned dice tomatoes

3 cups kale (chopped)

1/2 cup low-fat parmesan cheese (shredded)

Methods:

1. Drain and rinse the beans.

2. In a cooker, Tote up all the Constituents leaving the kale and parmesan. Cover the pot and cook and cook for 4 hours.

3. Tote up the kale and cook for another 30 min or until it is wilted.

4. Serve into serving bowls and it with parmesan cheese. Serve

Quinoa Vegan Meat Recipe

Prep Time: 15 min

Cook Time: 30 min

Total Time: 45 min

Serve: 5 cups

Nutrition Info: Calories: 91; Fiber: 2g| Total Fat: 3g | Carbs: 13g| Saturated Fat: 0g| Protein: 4g| Trans Fat: 0g| Sugar: 1g| Cholesterol: 0mg| Sodium: 163mg|

Constituents:

Vegan Meat Base

1 cup quinoa, rinsed

2 cups low-sodium vegetable broth

1/2 tsp black pepper

1/2 tsp salt

1 cup diced raw walnuts

3 tbsps tomato paste

1 tbsp yeast

Mexican Dishes

1/2 cup salsa

Garlic powder (1/4 tsp)

2 tsps chili powder

2 tsps cumin

Italian Dishes

1/2 cup marinara sauce

1/4 tsp garlic powder

2 tsps Italian seasoning or dried oregano

Methods:

1. To a pot, Tote up quinoa, vegetable broth, salt and pepper and allow boiling. Reduce the heat and cook until the broth is absorbed.

2. Turn off the heat and allow setting for 5 min.

3. Heat the oven to 400 degrees.

4. Tote up the other Constituents to the quinoa and stir well.

5. Spread the mixture evenly on a large parchment baking sheet.

6. Place in the oven and bake for 15 min. Stir again and bake for Tote up for additional 15 mins. Remove and enjoy.

Black Bean Lentil Soup

Prep Time: 10 mins

Cook Time: 40 mins

Total Time: 50 mins

Quota: 8 cups

Nutrition info:

Calories: 232; Fiber: 12g| Total Fat: 4g| Sugar: 3g| Saturated Fat: 3g| Sodium: 473mg| Trans Fat: 0g| Protein: 13g| Cholesterol: 0mg| Carbohydrates: 38g|

Constituents:

1/4 cup water

2 carrots, diced

1 sweet or yellow onion, diced

Canned diced tomatoes (14 1/2 oz)

1 cup green lentils, dry

30 ounce canned black beans

1 tsp cumin

1 tsp chili powder

Black pepper, (1/2 tsp)

Salt (1 tsp)

Red pepper flakes, crushed (1/8 tsp)

Vegetable broth-4 1/2 cups (You may also use water or a combination of both)

Coconut milk, canned (1/2 cup)

Methods:

1. Place a big pot over medium heat and Tote up water and sauté the diced onion.

2. Tote up the other Constituents, stir well and cover.

3. Let the soup boil and then decrease the heat.

4. Cook until carrots and lentils are tender.

Greek Lentil and Garlic Soup

Prep Time: 10 min

Cool Time: 35 min

Total Time: 45 min

Serve: 4

Nutrition Fact: Calories: 276; Sodium: 688mg| Carbs: 47g| Total Fat: 5g| Fiber: 9g| Saturated Fat: 1g | Protein: 15g| Trans Fat: 0g| Sugar: 5g| Cholesterol: 0mg

Constituents:

1 cup lentils, dry

1 tbsp olive oil

1/2 cup celery, diced small

Yellow onion (1 cup; diced small)

4 cloves garlic (minced)

1 cup carrot, diced

4 cups low-sodium vegetable broth

1 tsp ground rosemary

3 tsps dried oregano

2 bay leaves

1 tsp Kosher salt

1 tsp ground black pepper

4 tbsps no-sugar Tote up tomato paste

1 whole wheat pita

1 tbsp red wine vinegar

4 lemon wedges

Methods:

1. Bring a pot of water to boil. Rinse and Tote up the lentils to the boiling water.

2. Cook the lentils for 5 mins. Drain and set aside.

3. In a big sauce pan, heat olive oil.

4. In the hot oil, Tote up carrot, celery, onion and garlic. Cook until the onions are transparent.

5. Tote up the vegetable broth, rosemary, oregano, bay leaves and cooked lentils and allow boiling.

6. Reduce the heat and allow simmering for 20 min.

7. Remove the bay leaves from the simmering soup and Tote up 2 tbsps tomato paste. Stir well and simmer for Tote up for additional 5 mins.

8. Heat a skillet on medium heat and toast the pita lightly on each side. Remove and allow cooling.

9. Cut the pita into 8 parts.

10. Spoon soup into serving bowls and drizzle the red wine vinegar over each bowl. Squeeze lemon juice as desired.

11. Serve with pita toast and lemon wedge.

Quinoa Lentil and Mustard Burger

Prep Time: 10 min

Cook Time: 50 min

Total Time: 1 hour

Serve: 4

Nutritional Facts: Calories: 268 | Protein: 10 g| fiber: 9 g| Total Fat: 8 g | Sugars: 7 g| Saturated Fats: 1 g| Sodium: 679 mg Trans Fats: 0 g| Carbohydrates: 42 g| Cholesterol: 0 mg

Constituents:

Burger Recipe:

1 tbsp plus 2 tsps olive oil

1/4 cup diced red onion

1 cup cooked quinoa (cook according to manufacturer's Methods)

1 cup cooked brown lentils (well drained)

4 ounce can diced green chilies

1/3 cup rolled oats

White Whole Wheat Flour (1/4 cup)

2 tsps cornstarch

1/4 cup whole wheat panko bread crumbs

1/4 tsp garlic powder

1/2 tsp cumin

salt

Pepper

Honey Dijon Mustard Recipe

2 tbsps Dijon Mustard

3 tsps honey

Methods:

1. In 2 tsps olive oil, sauté the onion for about 4 min.

2. Prepare the Honey Dijon Mustard Recipe by cutting all the Constituents and refrigerating.

3. In a big bowl, combine all the burger Constituents and divide into 4 burger patties.

4. In a skillet, Tote up 1 tbsp olive oil and cook the patties until it is brown on both side.

5. Spread Honey Dijon Mustard (optional)

Grilled Spicy Tofu with Szechuan Veggies

Prep Time: 10 min

Cook Time: 54 min

Total Time: 1 hour 4 min

Serve: 4

Nutritional Info:

Calories: 297; Fiber: 5g| Total Fat: 20g | Protein: 24g|
Total Carbs: 14g| Saturated Fat: 3g| Trans Fat: 0g |
Sugars: 4g| Sodium: 84mg|

Constituents:

Tofu recipe:

1 pound firm tofu, frozen and thawed

1/4 tsp red pepper flakes

3 tbsps soy sauce (optional gluten-free Tamari)

2 tbsps toasted sesame oil

Apple cider vinegar (2 tbsps)

1 clove garlic, minced)

 Freshly grated ginger (1 tsp)

Vegetables:

Toasted sesame oil (1 tbsp)

1 pound fresh (trimmed) green beans

1 red bell pepper (sliced)

1 small red onion (sliced)

1 tsp soy sauce (optional gluten-free Tamari)

2 tbsps Szechuan sauce

1 tsp corn starch

Methods:

Tofu:

1. Cut the thawed tofu into half inch thick slices (square or triangle shape will do)

2. In a small bowl, Tote up the marinade Constituents.

3. Put the tofu in a baking dish and pour the marinade mixture over it.

4. Refrigerate for 40 minutes.

5. Heat your grill to medium heat and grill the tofu 5 minutes on each side until it is firm.

There should be grill marks on both sides

Vegetables:

1. In a pot, Tote up water and salt. Allow to boil and Tote up the green beans.

2. Blanch for 3 minutes. Drain and rinse the beans with cold water.

3. To a tsp of cold water, Tote up the corn starch.

4. Heat a big skillet over medium heat and Tote up the sesame oil followed by the green beans, red pepper and onions.

5. Tote up the Szechuan sauce and soy sauce and stir for 1 min.

6. Tote up the corn starch mixture to the vegetable and stir the mixture until it is thick. Serve the tofu with the vegetables.

Cleansing Vegetable Soup
Prep Time: 10 min

Cook Time: 7 hours 10 min

Total Time: 7 hours 10 min

Serve: 8

Nutrition Info: Calories: 152; Fiber: 7 g| Total Fat: 1 g | Sodium: 542 mg| Saturated Fat: 0 g | Protein: 9 g| carbohydrates: 29 g| Cholesterol: 0 mg| Sugars: 3 g| Trans Fat: 0 g

Constituents:

3 medium carrots, peeled and sliced

1 sweet potato, cut up into cubes

Celery, diced (1 stalk)

Yellow onion, diced

Garlic, minced (1 clove)

sea salt

Black pepper (1/2 tsp)

1/8 tsp allspice

Paprika (1 tsp)

1 bay leaf

2 (15 oz) cans navy beans

Vegetable broth, low-sodium (4 cups)

Optional Constituents:

14.5 oz. diced tomatoes

Olive oil- extra-virgin (1 tbsp plus 1 tsp)

Baby spinach, (4 cups)

Methods:

1. To a slow cooker, Tote up all the Constituents leaving out the spinach and olive oil.

2. Cook on low heat for 7 hours till vegetables are tender.

3. Tote up in the spinach, stir and continue cooking until wilted. Serve and enjoy.

Snacks

Easy To Make Stuffed Mushrooms Formula

Prep Time: 12 minutes

Cook Time: 22 minutes

Total Time: 34 minutes

Quota: 6

Nutritional Fact:

Calories: 146; Total Fat: 9 g| Carbs: 10 g| Saturated Fats: 4 g| Sugars: 4 g| Trans Fats: 0 g | Protein: 8 g| | Sodium: 215 mg| Cholesterol: 21 mg| Fiber: 2 g|

Constituents:

1 tbsp olive oil

12 baby Bella mushrooms (clean by patting with wet cloth, ensure not to use water)

1/2 Cup of Sliced sweet onion

2 Cloves of garlic (crushed)

1/4 Cup of sliced sun-dried tomatoes, wrapped up in olive oil

2 cups baby spinach, shredded into pieces

Panko bread crumbs (1/3 Cup)

4 ounce container feta cheese (low fat or fat free)

1/4 cup parmesan cheese

Methods:

1. Heat the oven to 350* degrees F.

2. Remove stems from the mushrooms and diced.

3. On low heat, put a skillet and add oil.

4. Sauté the onion, tomatoes and mushroom for 4 min.

5. Tote up the garlic and sauté for Tote up for additional one min.

6. Put in the spinach and sauté until wilted.

7. Set skillet down, Tote up the feta cheese, breadcrumbs and 3 tbsps parmesan cheese, stir.

8. Stuff the mushrooms with the mixture, place on a parchment pan and sprinkle the remaining parmesan.

9. Place pan into oven and heat until cheese has melted. Dish up while still warm.

Plant-Based- Cashew Bread

Prep Time: 12 mins

Cook Time: 30 mins

Total Time: 42 mins

Serves: 5

Nutritional Fact: Calories: 159; Fiber: 1 g| Sodium: 125 mg| Protein: 5 g| Saturated Fat: 2 g| Sugar: 2 g| Total Fat: 12 g| Cholesterol: 0 mg| Carbs: 10 g

Constituents:

Recipe for base

1 cup raw cashews

3/4 cup plus 1 tbsp water

2 cups water for soaking

Tote up for additional Constituents

1 tsp maple syrup

1/4 tsp black pepper

1/4 tsp salt

1/4 tsp garlic powder

1/2 tsp dried oregano

Methods:

1. First you heat up your oven to 400* degrees F and set up a baking dish with two parchment pieces then put aside.

2. Marinate the cashew in the water for 15 min. Rinse and drain well.

3. Tote up the drained cashew and the remaining water in a blender then blend till the result is a smooth pummel.

4. Tote up the other Constituents to the batter and blend it in.

5. Decant the muddle into the lined pan and spread evenly.

6. Cook for 15 mins in the oven, flip over and then bake for another 15 min.

7. Watch the bread to ensure it does not burn.

8. Flick, and leave it to chill on a rack before slicing.

Limed Cilantro With Three Bean Salad

Prep Time: 7 mins

Cook Time: 30 mins

Total Time: 37 mins

Serves: 6

Nutritional info: Calories: 308kcal | Saturated Fat: 1g| Total Fat: 7g| Sugar: 11g| Fiber: 11g| Cholesterol: 0mg |

Protein: 14g| | Carbohydrates: 49g| Trans Fat: 0g| Sodium: 525mg

Constituents:

15 ounce can of Cannellini beans, washed and dried

15 ounce can of Kidney beans, washed and drained

15 ounce can of Garbanzo beans, washed and drained

1/2 Red onion, nicely chopped

1/2 cup fresh and chopped cilantro

1/4 cup lime juice

2 tbsps olive oil

2 tbsps honey

1/2 tsp Kosher salt

1 tsp ground cumin

Methods:

1. In a large bowl, Tote up all Constituents and toss well.

2. Cover the mixture and refrigerate for 30 min or allow salad to sit overnight.

3. Toss again before serving.

Chia-Spiced Candied Nuts

Prep Time: 7 min

Cook Time: 15 min

Total Time: 22 min

Serves: 12

Nutrition Info: Calories: 213; Fiber: 2g| Total Fat: 19g| Carbohydrates: 10g| Sugar: 5g| Saturated Fat: 2g| Protein: 4g| Cholesterol: 0mg| Trans Fat: 0g| Sodium: 100mg|

Constituents:

1/2 tsp ground cardamom

1/8 tsp cayenne pepper

1 tsp ground cinnamon

Chia spice coating

3 tbsps real maple syrup

Nuts

1/2 tsp ginger powder

1/2 tsp sea salt

2 Tbsps of Olive oil (or melted coconut oil)

1 1/2 cups cashews

1 1/2 cups pecans

Methods:

1. Heat the oven to 350 degrees.

2. Whisk the chia spice coating and all other Constituents except the nuts.

3. Cover the nuts in the mix till it is well-coated.

4. Spread out the nuts evenly in a non-sticking pan and then roast for 15 min.

5. Take care to stir the nuts every 5 min during the cook time.

6. When the nuts are golden in color, remove from the oven and enjoy.

Vegan Avocado Wontons

Prep Time: 10 min

Cook Time: 20 min

Total Time: 30 min

Serves: 6

Nutrition info: Calories: 265; Fiber: 4g| Sodium: 467mg| Total Fat: 8g| Sugar: 0g| Saturated Fat: 1g| Trans Fat: 0g| Carbohydrates: 41g| Cholesterol: 6mg| Protein: 7g

Constituents:

1 avocado, large

1/2 tbsp chopped cilantro

1 tsp rice vinegar

1 tsp sesame oil

1 large avocado

1/2 cup shredded coleslaw veggies mix

2 tsps soy sauce (optional)

12 wonton wrappers

Methods:

1. Pre-heat the oven to 400 degrees.

2. Put the avocado, sesame oil, soy sauce, cilantro, coleslaw and rice vinegar, together and mash well.

3. Into each wonton wrapper, spoon 1 tbsp of the mixture.

4. Use your finger to run it along the edges of the wrapper (after dipping it in water).

5. crease the wrapper crossways and tweak the edges together.

6. Line a baking sheet and place the wantons.

7. Cook for10 mins in the oven.

8. Flip over and bake the other side for another 10 minutes.

9. Dish up with soy sauce or eat plain.

Vegan Sunflower Lentil Dip

Prep Time: 10 Mins

Cook Time: 7 Mins

Total Time: 17 Mins

Serve: 16

Nutrition Info: Calories: 100; Carbs: 16g| Fiber: 3g| Total Fat: 2g| Protein: 6g| Sodium: 68mg| Saturated Fat: 0g | Cholesterol: 0mg| Sugar: 1g| Trans Fat: 0g

Constituents:

2 cups red lentils, cooked until tender

1 tbsp lemon juice

1/2 tsp salt

1/4 tsp pepper

Garlic, crushed (2 cloves)

1 tbsp of olive oil

2 tbsps sunflower seeds

2 tbsps celery, (diced)

1 tbsp red onion, (diced)

1 tbsp fresh tarragon, (minced)

2 tbsps fresh parsley, (minced)

Methods:

1. Tote up the lemon juice, pepper, salt, olive oil and lentil in a blender and blend until smooth.

2. Tote up the remaining Constituents and stir.

3. Enjoy with fresh vegetables or wheat pita.

Quinoa and Lentils Meatballs
Prep Time: 10 min

Cook Time: 30 min

Total Time: 40 min

Quota: 6

Nutritional info: Calories: 291 | Fiber: 6 g| Protein: 13 g| Sodium: 309 mg| Trans Fats: 0 g| Cholesterol: 3 mg| Carbohydrates: 39 g| Sugars: 2 g| Saturated Fats: 2 g| Total Fat: 10 g

Constituents:

½ cup dry quinoa, (rinsed)

1 cup water

Cooked green lentils (1 Cup) and sapped out

¼ cup of chopped red bell pepper

½ cup of sliced onion

2 cloves garlic, (minced)

½ cup of gluten-free bread crumbs or whole wheat panko bread crumbs

¼ cup of freshly ground parmesan

1 tbsp of freshly chopped flat parsley leaves

1 tbsp freshly chopped oregano

1/2 tsp of freshly grated black pepper

Sea salt

¼ tsp of Cayenne pepper

1 egg white

3 tbsps olive oil

Methods:

1. Place a pot on a stove and Tote up water and quinoa. Allow to boil. Decrease the heat and leave it to bubble for 15 mins.

2. Take it off the heat and leave it to cool. Press quinoa with a paper towel to empty extra water.

3. In a bowl, combine all the Constituents except the oil. Mix well.

4. Mash the Constituents until the lentils are mashed as well.

5. Mould the mixture into small meatball using your hands. Refrigerate for 2 hours.

6. Put a skillet on medium heat, Tote up the olive hot and cook the meatballs.

7. Cook the balls till they get browned. Flip over and cook as well.

8. Remove and drain using a paper towel.

Spicy Mango Salsa

Prep Time: 12 mins

Cook Time: 10 min

Total Time: 22 min

Serve: 4 cups

Nutrition Info:

Calories: 32; Sodium: 121mg| Protein: 1g| Trans Fat: 0g|
Sugar: 6g| Total Fat: 0g| Carbohydrates: 7g| Fiber: 1g|
Cholesterol: 0mg| Saturated Fat: 0g

Constituents:

1 medium mango, peeled, pit removed, and diced small

1 jalapeno, (minced)

1 tbsp of lime juice

1 tbsp fresh cilantro, (chopped)

1/2 tsp of Kosher salt

6 Roma tomatoes, (diced small)

1 small red onion, (diced small)

1 small and sliced red bell pepper

51/4 tsp ground cumin

Methods:

1. Combine tomato, onion, mango, pepper and jalapeno and mix well. Tote up the remainder of the Components then toss.

2. Leave it to rest for10 min before you serve.

Spinach and Artichoke Dip Recipe

Prep Time:

Cook Time:

Total Time:

Serves: 6

Nutrition info:

Calories: 70; Fiber: 3.0 g| Sodium: 658 mg| Saturated Fat: 0 g| Protein: 5.5 g| Cholesterol: 0 mg| Total Fat: 2.0 g| Carbohydrates: 8.3 g| Trans Fat: 0 g| Sugars: 1.9 g

Constituents:

1 tbsp of freshly squashed lemon juice

1 1/2 tsp kosher salt

1/2 tsp of freshly grated black pepper

1 small onion

4 garlic cloves

6-ounce jar of quartered artichoke hearts

12.3 ounce packaged low-fat silken tofu

10-ounce package frozen chopped spinach, (thawed)

Pinch of cayenne pepper

Methods:

1. Heat up the oven to 350* degrees F.

2. Using an aluminum foil, wrap the garlic and onion.

3. Cook for 30 mins in the oven.

4. Place spinach in a dish towel and squeeze to wring out the surplus water as possible.

5. Blend the onion, garlic, artichokes and well drained spinach in a blender. Tote up in the remaining Constituents and blend until smooth.

Chocolate and Peanut Butter Bites

Prep Time: 20 min

Total Time: 20 min

Serve: 20

Nutrition Info:

Calories: 94; Trans Fat: 0g| Protein: 3g| Carbs: 12g|
Cholesterol: 0mg| Fiber: 2g| Sodium: 2mg| Total Fat: 5g|
Sugars: 5g| Saturated Fat: 1g

Constituents:

1/8 tsp kosher or sea salt

1/4 cup flax seeds (any variety)

1/4 cup (unsweetened) cocoa powder

1/2 cup natural creamy peanut butter

3 tbsps chia seeds

1 cup old fashioned rolled oats

1/3 cup honey (or real maple syrup)

1 tsp real vanilla extract

Methods:

1. Grind half cup oats and all the flax seeds to powder in a blender.

2. Tote up the powder, remaining oat, salt, cocoa powder and chia seeds in a bowl and mix.

3. In a separate bowl, combine the vanilla extract, peanut butter and honey.

4. Tote up the honey mixture to the dry Constituents and stir thoroughly. Roll up into small balls about 20 balls.

5. Remember to wet hands with water or coconut oil to prevent mixture from sticking to your hands.

Desserts

Banana Pudding Cream

Prep Time: 5 min

Total Time: 5 min

Serves: 2

Nutrition info:

Calories: 249; Cholesterol: 0mg| Sugar: 19g| Total Fat: 11g| Fiber: 5g| Saturated Fat: 1g| Trans Fat: 0g| Carbs: 37g| Protein: 6g| sodium: 33mg

Constituents:

2 large ripe bananas cut into small pieces, (freeze for 12 hours)

1/2 cup (unsweetened) almond milk

1/4 cup chopped walnuts

Methods:

1. Blend almond milk in a blender, then Tote up the banana pieces until puree.

2. Top with walnuts and serve.

Avocado and Banana Brownie Formula

Prep Time: 15 min

Cook Time: 30 min

Total Time: 45 min

Ration: 12 pieces

Nutrition Info:

Calories: 240; Saturated Fat: 3g| Cholesterol: 0mg| Sugar: 6g| Protein: 8g| Fiber: 6g| Sodium: 7mg| Carbohydrates: 23g| Total Fat: 16g| Trans Fat: 0g

Constituents:

3 large overly ripe bananas

1 medium ripe avocado

1 cup of Crunchy peanut butter

Vanilla (1 tsp)

1/2 cup of raw powder

1/4 cup of almond flour (or meal)

 Millet (/2 Cup)

1/4 cup of cocoa nibs

1/2 cup walnut pieces, (optional)

Methods:

1. Set oven to 359* F degrees.

2. Using a fork, mash avocado and banana together. You should have 2 cups after mashing.

3. Stir in peanut butter and vanilla. Combine well.

4. Fold in the cacao, millet almond meal, cocoa powder and nibs and walnuts (optional).

5. Mix all Constituents well and pour in a parchment lined baking pan

6. Bake until the top is no longer wet.

7. Cool the brownie completely and refrigerate for 3 hours before cutting.

Vegan No-Bake Cookie chocolate coated dough Bars

Prep Time: 15 minutes

Total Time: 15 minutes

Serve: 10 bars

Nutrition Info:

Calories: 316; Fiber: 5g| Protein: 6g| Trans Fat: 0g|
Sodium: 56mg| Saturated Fat: 6g| Carbs: 32g| Sugar:
22g| Total Fat: 21g| Cholesterol: 0mg

Constituents:

Cookie Dough:

1 cup almond flour

1/3 cup pure maple syrup

1/3 cup almond butter

1/2 tsp vanilla extract

3/4 cup of chocolate chips (semi-sweet)

2 tbsps coconut flour

1/4 tsp Kosher salt

For the Chocolate topping:

1 cup semisweet Vegan chocolate chips

2 tbsps almond butter

Methods:

Cookie Dough:

1. Prepare a baking sheet and spray with nonstick spray.

2. Mix all the Constituents except the chips. Then fold in
the chips carefully.

3. Spread the mixture on the prepared tin and press onto the pan evenly. Refrigerate it until it is pretty firm.

4. Finish with chocolate topping before serving. Serve and enjoy.

Chocolate toppings:

1. Melt the almond butter and chocolate chips together until smooth. Pour over the melted mixture over the frozen bars and serve.

Vegetarian Caramel Apple Parfait

Prep Time: 10 Mins

Cook Time: 15 Mins

Total Time: 25 Mins

Serves: 4

Nutrition info:

Calories: 259 | Sodium: 63 mg| Trans Fat: 0 g| Carbohydrates: 21 g| Cholesterol: 0 mg| Protein: 5 g|

Fiber: 6 g| Total Fat: 18 g| Sugar: 11 g| Saturated Fat: 9 g|

Constituents:

2 cups almond milk

1/4 cup chia seeds

1 tsp of grated cinnamon

1/4 cup of liquefied coconut oil

1/4 cup pure maple syrup

2 tbsps almond butter

1/2 cup apples, (peeled, cored and diced)

Methods:

1. Put and mix together in a bowl, the chia seeds, coconut milk and grated cinnamon.

2. cover and freeze for an hr.

2. To make the vegan caramel, Tote up the almond butter, maple syrup, and coconut oil in a bowl and beat well until smooth.

3. clinch the bowl with a wrap (plastic) till you are set to dish up.

Spiced Carrot Oatmeal Cookies

Prep Time: 10 Mins

Cook Time: 15 Mins

Total Time: 25 Mins

Serve: 12 Cookies

Nutrition Info:

Calories: 181; Sodium: 69mg| Sugar: 13g| Trans Fat: 0g|
Protein: 4g| Carbohydrates: 31g| Fiber: 3g| Total Fat: 5g|
Saturated Fat: 4g| cholesterol: 0mg

Constituents:

1 cup oats

3/4 cup whole wheat flour

Baking powder (1 1/2 tsp)

Cinamon, ground (1 tsp)

1/2 cup coconut milk

1/2 cup applesauce

1 tsp almond extract

1/2 tsp ground cloves

2 tbsps coconut oil, (melted)

1 cup granulated coconut sugar

1 cup carrots, (grated)

Methods:

1. Set oven to 325 *degree F and prepare a baking sheet.

2. In a clean bowl, Tote up oats, baking powder, cinnamon, clove and flour together. Mix.

3. In a bowl, mix the coconut milk, almond extract, coconut oil and sugar. Fold in the flour mixture gradually.

4. Take care to mix well. Tote up the carrots.

5. Using a Tbsp, scoop the batter to the all set-up baking sheet.

6. Cook for 10 min in the oven and let it chill a bit before you dish up.

Peppermint Fudge Formula

Prep Time: 5 min

Cook Time: 7 min

Total Time: 12 min

Serve: 20

Nutritional Facts:

Calories: 143 g; Sodium: 35 mg| Protein: 1 g| Trans Fat: 0 g| Fiber: 1 g| Sugars: 14 g| Carbs: 17 g| Total Fat: 10 g| Cholesterol: 0 mg| Saturated Fat: 5 g

Constituents:

2 1/2 cups chocolate chips

a dash of kosher or sea salt

Pure peppermint extract (1 tsp)

1/2 cup walnuts (diced, optional)

1/3 cup canned coconut milk

1/4 cup of coconut palm sugar

1 tbsp pure butter (or coconut oil)

Methods:

1. Stir chocolate chips, coconut milk, butter or coconut oil, sugar and coconut milk in a saucepan.

2. Put saucepan on low heat and leave the chocolate to melt totally. Stir well to prevent from burning.

3. Take pan off the heat after the chocolate has melted and tote up the pepper mint.

4. Tote up the walnuts if using and stir.

5. Cool the fudge to room temperature.

6. Grease a casserole dish & decant the fudge into it.

7. Refrigerate until it is set. Cut the fudge into 30 squares.

Nutty Banana Chocolate Bread

Prep Time: 12 mins

Cook Time: 60 mins

Total Time: 72 mins

Serve: 8

Nutritional info:

Calories: 293; Fiber: 6 g| Protein: 6 g| Carbohydrates: 62 g| Trans Fat: 0 g| Sodium: 144 mg| Total Fat: 5 g| | Sugars: 33 g| Cholesterol: 0 mg| Saturated Fat: 2 g

Constituents:

4-5 overly ripe bananas

1/4 cup cocoa powder

1/2 tsp of baking soda

Cinnamon (tsp)

1 cup coconut palm sugar

1/4 cup water

1 tsp vanilla

1 3/4 cup whole wheat flour

1/4 cup of vegan chocolate chips

1/4 cup of nuts (diced walnuts & pecans)

Baking powder (1 tsp)

Methods:

1. Set oven to 350*degrees F.

2. In a large clean bowl, mash the ripe bananas and Tote up the vanilla and coconut palm sugar. Using a hand mixer, mix well and Tote up water during mixing.

3. Mix the other Constituents except the chips in another bowl. Tote up the mixed dry Constituents to the wet contents and mix fully with a spatula.

4. Crease in the nuts & chips.

5. Scoop the pound into a bake pan and cook for 1 hr.

Lemony Cranberry Cheesecake-Vegan

Prep Time: 10 min

Total Time: 10 min

Serve: 24 squares

Nutrition info:

Calories: 262; Protein: 5 g| Sodium: 50 mg| Fiber: 3 g| Cholesterol: 0 mg| Total Fat: 23 g| Carbs: 11 g| Saturated Fat: 10 g| Sugars: 3 g| Trans Fat: 0 g

Constituents:

Crust Constituents:

2 cups raw almonds

2 cups chopped pitted dates

1/2 cup raw cacao powder

Filling Constituents:

3 cups raw cashews soaked for 2 hours

1 cup organic unrefined coconut oil

3/4 cup raw agave

1/2 cup fresh lemon juice

Water (1/2 cup)

1 tbsp of lemon zest

1 tsp of alcohol free vanilla extract

a pinch Celtic sea salt

Methods:

Crust:

1. Combine the dates, almonds and cocoa powder using a food processor.

2. Roll up into a ball.

3. Oil a baking tin using coconut oil.

4. Press the crust down in the pan and keep aside.

Filling:

1. Place all the filling Constituents into a processor and blend it until creamy. Pour into the crust tin.

2. Seal tin with foil (aluminum) & refrigerate for 10 hrs.

3. Remember to defrost the cake and place in the fridge for 1 hr before you dish up.

Coconut and Mango Ice Cream

Prep Time: 7 min

Total Time: 7 min

Serve: 6

Nutrition Info:

Calories: 189; Sodium: 8 mg| Fiber: 2 g| Saturated Fat: 7 g| Carbohydrates: 30 g| Protein: 2 g| Total Fat: 9 g| Dietary| Sugars: 26 g| Trans Fat: 0 g| Cholesterol: 0mg

Constituents:

1 cup canned coconut milk (full-fat recommended)

3 cups organic mango (diced and frozen)

1 tbsp honey (optional)

Methods:

1. In a blender, put the mango, honey, and coconut milk and blend until a soft ice cream consistency.

2. Devour!

Vegan Strawberry Banana Bread

Prep Time: 6 min

Cook Time: 17 min

Total Time: 25 min

Serve: 24 mini loaves

Nutrition info:

Calories: 87; Saturated Fat: 2 g| Protein: 1 g| Sodium: 55 mg| Trans Fat: 0 g| Total Fat: 3 g| Carbohydrates: 15 g| Fiber: 1 g| Cholesterol: 0 mg| Sugars: 7 g|

Constituents:

1 cup over-ripe bananas (mashed)

2 1/2 tbsps of chia seeds

Coconut oil, softened (1 Tbsp)

1 tbsp of vanilla

Coconut milk (2/3 Cup)

3 tbsps of maple syrup

2 1/2 tsps baking powder

1 1/4 cup gluten-free flour blend

1 tbsp cinnamon

Methods:

1. Set oven to 350*degrees F.

2. Beat the maple syrup, coconut milk, banana, coconut oil, vanilla and chia seeds in a bowl. Allow it to rest for 5 min.

3. Mix the baking powder, flour and cinnamon. Fold the flour mixture into the wet Constituents. Mix well.

4. Tote up the strawberries.

5. Using nonstick spray, spray a 24- mini loaf tin and split the pummel into the tin.

6. Bake in the oven for 12 min.

Oil-Free chocolate Muffin Recipe

Prep Time: 10 min

Cook Time: 30 min

Total Time: 40 min

Serve: 12

Nutritional Facts:

Calories: 105; Sodium: 100mg | Cholesterol: 0mg|
Carbohydrates: 23g| Protein: 5g| Saturated Fat: 1g| Fiber:
6g| Sugar: 10g| Trans Fat: 0g| Total Fat: 1g

Constituents:

1 3/4 cup of cooked black beans

1 small banana

1/4 cup (unsweetened) applesauce

6 tbsps water

2 (helpful) tbsps ground flax seed

3/4 cup (raw, organic) cacao powder

1/2 (heap full) cup coconut palm sugar

1 1/2 tsp of baking powder

Arrowroot powder (1 tsp)

1 tsp of vanilla extract

Salt (/4 tsp)

Methods:

1. Set oven to 350*degrees F.

2. Blend all Constituents to a puree in a processor.

3. Clean a muffin tin (12-cup) & pour the puree uniformly.

4. Bake the mixture for 30 min.

5. Allow the muffin to chill then you dish up.

Smoothies

Avocado and Pear Smoothie

Prep Time: 5 min

Total Time: 5 min

Serve: 2

Nutrition Info:

Calories: 272; Sugars: 29 g| Sodium: 124 mg| Protein: 10 g| Trans Fat: 0 g| Carbohydrates: 38 g| Saturated Fat: 3 g| Fiber: 6 g| Total Fat: 10 g| Cholesterol: 12 mg

Constituents:

2 tsps raw honey

1/4 tsp vanilla extract

Ice

1/2 cup non-fat plain Greek yogurt

1/2 ripe avocado, (peeled and pitted)

1 ripe pear, (cored and chopped)

Directions:

1. Using a blender, blend all Constituents until it is smooth.

Blue Paradise and Pineapple Smoothie

Prep Time: 7 min

Total Time: 7 min

Serve: 2

Nutrition info:

Calories: 201; Fiber: 3 gm | Saturated Fats: 4 gm | Protein: 9 gm | Total Fat: 6 gm | Sodium: 61 mg | Carbs: 29 gm | Cholesterol: 4 mg | Sugars: 22 gm | Trans Fats: 0 gm

Constituents:

1/2 cup frozen unsweetened pineapple chunks (about 8)

Frozen wild blueberries (1 cup)

1/2 cup plain fat free Greek Yogurt

2 cups organic baby spinach

1/2 cup light coconut milk (organic or skimmed milk)

1/2 cup unsweetened pineapple juice

Methods:

1. Using a food processor, blend all the Constituents until it is smooth.

Super Smoothie

Prep Time: 10 min

Total Time: 10 min

Quota: 3

Nutritional Facts:

Calories: 131; Fiber: 4 g| Sugars: 13 g| Protein: 7 g| saturated fat: 0g| Carbohydrates: 26 g| Trans Fat: 0 g| sodium: 287mg| Total Fat: 1 g| Cholesterol: 2 mg

Constituents:

1 cup of organic baby spinach and loosely packed

Frozen banana (1 small) slice before you freeze

Frozen berries (1 cup) and unsweetened

Fresh ginger root (1/2 slice)

1/2 cup of kefir of Greek yoghurt plain low-fat

1 cup of unsweetened chilled green tea

Pure pomegranate juice (1/2 cup)

Crushed ice (1 cup)

Methods:

1. Blend all Constituents in a blender until it is smooth. You can Tote up green tea to make the smoothie thinner.

Super Blast Smoothie

Prep Time: 5 min

Total Time: 5 min

Quota: 3

Nutrition Fact:

Calories: 130; Sodium: 23 mg| Fiber: 3 gm| Saturated Fats: 0 gm| Sugars: 21 gm| Trans Fats: 0 gm| Protein: 5 gm| Cholesterol: 2 mg| Total Fat: 1 gm| Carbohydrates: 27 gm|

Constituents:

1/2 cup chilled green tea, (unsweetened)

1 tbsp honey (optional)

1 organic (sweet) apple, cored and peeled

1 cup (frozen) red grapes

1 tsp freshly grated ginger

1/2 cup kefir, plain

1/2 cup chilled green tea, (unsweetened)

1 tbsp honey (optional)

ice cubes

Methods:

1. Blend all the constituents in a processor until smooth.

Immune Booster Vegan Smoothie

Prep Time: 5 min

Total Time: 5 min

Serve: 2

Nutrition info:

Calories: 156; Sodium: 287 mg| Fiber: 4 g| Trans Fat: 0 g|
Protein: 10 g| Cholesterol: 2 mg| Total Fat: 3 g|
Carbohydrates: 26 g| Sugars: 13 g | Saturated Fat: .5 g

Constituents:

1 frozen sliced banana

1 knuckle ginger root

1/2 avocado, (peeled)

1 cup red kale (organic if possible)

1/8 tsp cinnamon

1 cup of organic froze red grapes

Coconut fresh meat (1/4 cup)

1/4 cup of pomegranate seeds

1 cup of baby spinach (organic if feasible)

Unsweetened chilled green tea (1 1/2 cups)

Ice cubes

Methods:

1. Blend all the Constituents in a processor until it is smooth and creamy.

Ever-young Smoothie
Prep Time: 7 Mins

Total Time: 7 Mins

Serve: 4 servings

Nutrition Facts:

Calories: 162; Fiber: 6g| Carbs: 22g| Trans Fat: 0g| Protein: 4g| Cholesterol: 1mg| Saturated Fat: 2g| Sodium: 36mg| Total Fat: 8g| Sugars: 11g|

Constituents:

1 peeled-kiwi

1 Cp of chopped green kale and the stems detached

Honeydew melon 1/8 and chopped to around 10 (inch) cubes

1 frozen banana

Baby spinach (1 cup)

1 peeled & seeded avocado

Low-fat milk; Soy or almond will do fine (about sss1/2 Cup)

Method:

1. Blend all the constituents in a blender until smooth and then Tote up extra milk to make the texture thinner.

Banana Ginger and Pomegranate Mishmash

Prep Time: 12 Mins

Total Time: 12 Mins

Serve: 2

Nutrition Facts:

Calories: 195; Fiber: 3 g| Protein: 8 g| Saturated Fat: 1 g| Carbohydrates: 39 g| Cholesterol: 7 | Sugars: 28 g| Sodium: 89 mg| Total Fat: 2 g |Trans Fat: 0 g

Constituents:

1 frozen Banana (ensure to slice before you freeze)

1/2 Cup of fat-free plain Greek yogurt

1/4 of a Knuckle Ginger Root (knuckle means the length of the joint of a finger)

Pure Pomegranate juice (1 Cup) and no sugar Tote up

Ice cubes about 4-5

Methods:

1. Blend all the components till it gets smooth.

Quinoa Raspberry Smoothie
Prep Time: 5 min

Total Time: 5 min

Serve: 2

Nutrition Info:

Calories: 141; Protein: 4 g| Cholesterol: 0 mg| Fiber: 7 g| Carbohydrates: 30 g| Saturated Fat: 0 g| Sodium: 6 mg| Sugars: 10 g| Total Fat: 1 g| Trans Fat: 0 g

Constituents:

1 cup frozen raspberries

1 1/2 cups green tea

6 ice cubes

1/2 cup cooked Quinoa (chill it)

1 frozen banana (pre-sliced)

Methods:

1. Blend all the listed Constituents until smooth; using a blender.

Peanut Butter Cum Banana Mishmash

Prep Time: 5 min

Total Time: 5 min

Quota: 2

Nutrition Facts:

Calories: 173; Fiber: 5 g| Protein: 12 g| Fat: 6 g| Sugar: 11 g| Sodium: 130 g| Carbs: 20 g|

Constituents:

1 banana, frozen (slice before freezing)

Peanut butter (about 1 Tbsp)

Protein powder (1 serving spoon)

Almond milk; plain and 1 1/2 Cups

Methods:

1. Blend all the listed Constituents until it is smooth and then mix in ice for a better texture.

Mediterranean Organic Smoothie
Prep Time: 5 mins

Cook Time: 5 mins

Total Time: 10 mins

Serves: 2

Nutritional Facts:

Calories: 168; Sodium: 69 mg| Saturated Fat: 1 g| Cholesterol: 2 mg| Sugars: 29 g| Carbohydrates: 39| Protein: 4 g| Fiber: 5 g| Total Fatt: 1 g| Trans fat: 0

Constituents:

2 cups loosely packed organic baby spinach

1 tsp fresh minced ginger root

1 frozen banana (pre-sliced)

1 small mango

1/2 cup beet juice

1/2 cup skimmed milk (unsweetened almond milk)

6 ice cubes

Methods:

1. Blend all the listed constituents till is smooth.

Sunrise Smoothie
Prep Time: 30 min

Total Time: 30 min

Serve: 3

Calories: 76; Trans Fat: 0 g| Protein: 1 g| Cholesterol: 0 mg| Sugars: 14 g| Fiber: 2 g| Carbohydrates: 17 g| Sodium: 27 mg| Total Fat: 1 g| Saturated Fat: 0 g

Constituents:

1 cup (frozen) mangoes

1/2 cup freshly-squeezed orange juice

Frozen strawberries (1 cup)

1/2 cup almond milk

Methods:

1. Combine the almond milk & strawberry in a blender and blend until it is smooth.

2. Pour the smoothie into 3 glasses and refrigerate for 20 min.

3. Blend the orange juice and mango until it is smooth and pour in the refrigerated glasses. Dish up ASAP!

Strawberry and Goji Berry Cumbo

Prep Time: 20 min

Total Time: 20 min

Serve: 2

Nutrition Info:

Calories: 197; Sodium: 147 mg| Fiber: 2 g| Saturated Fat: 3 g| Protein: 3 g| Trans Fat: 0 g| Carbohydrates: 30 g| Cholesterol: 18| Sugars: 21 g| Total Fat: 5 g

Constituents:

1 cup strawberries, hulled

2 tsps honey, optional

2 tbsps dried Goji berries

2 cups almond milk (or low-fat milk)

Ice cube

1 tbsp water

Methods:

1. In a clean bowl, Tote up water and Goji berries and to rest for 15 min.

2. Using a food processor, blend the soft Goji berry and other Constituents until they become smooth.

Minty Blueberry and Flax Seed Smoothie

Prep Time: 5 min

Total Time: 5 min

Serve: 2

Nutrition info:

Calories: 200; Protein: 10 g| Fiber: 2 g| Saturated Fat: 3 g|
Trans Fat: 0 g| Total Fat: 7 g| Carbohydrates: 26 g|
Sodium: 136 mg| Sugars: 23 g| g| Cholesterol: 18 mg

Constituents:

1/4 cup blueberries, (fresh or frozen)

1 tbsp honey (if using unsweetened use almond milk)

1 tbsp of flax seeds

2 cups of chilled almond milk (or dairy milk)

Methods:

1. Blend all the Constituents until it is smooth in a food
processor.

Mango & Basil Smoothie

Prep Time:

Total Time:

Serve: 2 servings

Nutrition Info:

Calories: 260; Fiber: 3 g| Trans Fat: 0 g| Protein: 12 g|
Cholesterol: 18 mg| Total Fat: 6 g| Sodium: 56 mg|
Carbohydrates: 43 g| Saturated Fatt: 3 g| Sugars: 34 g|

Constituents:

Honey (if almond milk is unsweetened)

1/2 tsp cinnamon powder

4 medium of fresh basil leaves

2 tbsps old fashioned oats

1 ripe mango, pitted and peeled

2 cups of almond milk or (dairy milk)

Methods:

1. Blend the oats to powder using a blender.

2. Put in the rest of the Constituents and blend until it is smooth.

Skinny Banana Split Protein Smoothie

Prep Time: 7 min

Total Time: 7 min

Serve: 2

Nutrition Info:

Calories: 217; Fiber: 3 g| Trans Fat: 0 g| Protein: 17 g| Saturated Fat: 1 g| Sodium: 150 mg| Carbohydrates: 29 g| Sugars: 19 g| Total Fat: 4 g| Cholesterol: 8 mg

Constituents:

1/2 cup non-fat Greek yogurt

1/2 cup (unsweetened) almond milk (can be replaced with other kinds of low-fat milk)

1 tbsp (unsalted) almonds

1/2 cup strawberries, (hulled and rinsed)

1 banana, (peeled and sliced)

2 scoops protein powder (clean)

Ice cubes

Methods:

1. Blend all the Constituents except the ice until smooth.

2. Tote up ice cubes and blend again till it becomes smooth. Serve smoothie right away.

Mango and Orange Smoothie Diet

Prep Time: 5 min

Total Time: 5 min

Serve: 2 smoothies

Nutrition info:

Calories: 320; Sugars: 56 g| Fiber: 4 g| Cholesterol: 11 mg| Saturated Fat: 0 g| Carbohydrates: 62 g| Sodium: 30 mg| Total Fat: 0 g| Protein: 12 g| Trans Fat: 0 g|

Constituents:

2 cups mango chunks (frozen)

1-1/2 cups non-fat Greek yogurt

1/2 tsp real vanilla extract

1-1/2 cups natural orange juice

1-1/2 cups crushed ice

Methods:

1. In a food processor, Tote up the yogurt, juice, ice and mango chunks and blend until it is smooth.

2. Serve into drinking glasses.

Vegan Pumpkin Spice Smoothie

Prep Time: 5 min

Total Time: 5 min

Serve: 2

Nutrition Info:

Calories: 138; Fiber: 2 g| Protein: 5 g| Cholesterol: 9 mg|
Saturated Fat: 1 g| Total Fat: 2 g| Carbohydrates: 25 g|
Sodium: 69 mg| Sugars: 18 g| Constituents:

1 tbsp pure maple syrup

1/4 tsp vanilla

1/4 tsp cinnamon

1/2 cup pumpkin puree, (canned or fresh)

1 frozen banana

1 cup almond milk, (or soy, lite coconut or skimmed milk)

1/8 tsp nutmeg

1/8 tsp allspice

1/2 cup ice

Methods:

1. blend all the components in a blender till is well
integrated.

Apple and Coconut Smoothie

Prep Time:

Total Time:

Quota: 2

Nutrition Info:

Calories: 185; Fiber: 5 g| Trans Fat: 0 g| Protein: 5g Total Fat: 5 g| Sodium: 74 mg| Carbohydrates: 33 g| Sugars: 22 g| Saturated Fat: 3 g| Cholesterol: 10 mg

Constituents:

1 cup baby spinach

1/2 tsp ground cinnamon

1 cup ice cubes

1 cup coconut milk

1 Granny Smith apple, (chopped)

1 banana

Methods:

1. In a food processor, Tote up all the Constituents and blend until it is creamy. Serve the smoothie immediately.

Razzle-Dazzle Smoothie-Vegan

Prep Time: 2 min

Total Time: 2min

Serve: 2 cups

Nutritional Info:

Calories: 180; Sodium: 85 mg| Sugars: 22 gm| Saturated Fats: 0 gm| Protein: 10 gm| Fiber: 5 gm| Cholesterol: 5 mg| Carbohydrates: 35 gm| Total Fat: 1 g| Trans Fats: 0 gm

Constituents:

1 medium Gala apple, (sliced)

1/2 cup fat free plain Greek Yogurt

1/2 cup skimmed milk

1/2 cup

1 cup kale, (stems removed and chopped)

1 cup baby spinach (loosely packed)

1 frozen banana, (sliced)

Methods:

1. In a blender, place all the Constituents and blend until it is creamy.

2. Pour into drinking glasses and Tote up a little cinnamon.

END

Thank you for reading my book. If you enjoyed it, won't you please take a moment to write a good review about my book and recommend it your friends and family?

Thanks!

Helen Kingsley